This book belongs to:

_____

my Body & Me

RECLAIMING THE
HEALTH
YOU DESERVE

SUSANNE RIDOLFI

My Body and Me: Reclaiming the H - E - A - L - T - H You Deserve
© Susanne Ridolfi 2022

www.susanneridolfi.com

The moral rights of Susanne Ridolfi to be identified as the author of this work has been asserted in accordance with the Copyright Act 1968.

First published in Australia 2022 by Susanne Ridolfi

ISBN 978-0-6455682-0-2

Any opinions expressed in this work are exclusively those of the author and are not necessarily the views held or endorsed by Susanne Ridolfi.

All rights reserved. No part of this publication may be reproduced or transmitted by any means, electronic, photocopying or otherwise, without prior written permission of the author.

Disclaimer

All the information, techniques, skills, and concepts contained within this publication are of the nature of general comment only and are not in any way recommended as individual advice. The intent is to offer a variety of information to provide a wider range of choices now and in the future, recognising that we all have widely diverse circumstances and viewpoints. Should any reader choose to make use of the information herein, this is their decision, and the author and publisher/s do not assume any responsibilities whatsoever under any conditions or circumstances. The author does not take responsibility for the business, financial, personal, or other success, results, or fulfilment upon the readers' decision to use this information. It is recommended that the reader obtain their own independent advice.

Dedicated to my parents – two loving souls always encouraging me to
Be and Do Me

Foreword

With the endless list of demands that modern life places on us, it is more important than ever to prioritise our health and wellbeing: to listen to what our body is saying and to form a deep connection with our true home on Earth.

I learned this when I was just 30 years old. I had worked myself into the ground in my business. I was overweight, wound-up, and anxious. My hormones were out of balance, I had leaky gut, and I was exhausted. It took months of focused healing to recover. To this day, I am grateful for the inspiration Susanne provided me on my journey of reclaiming my wellness.

Susanne encourages us to do what we know is right for our body – and give ourselves the care that is not a luxury, but a *necessity*.

We cannot perform in our lives, careers, relationships, and financial life if we are neglecting the critical relationship with our body. But when we embrace and nourish our body – through the principles and extensive knowledge Susanne has shared in this book – we can thrive as women.

Susanne lives and breathes her wisdom, and her own glowing well-being is proof of the power of her teachings. Just by being who she is, Susanne encourages us to take care of ourselves – body, mind, and soul.

I know her heartfelt desire is to see thousands more women around the world enjoying the incredible energy, radiance, and wellness that is possible for each one of us. This book is an important part of this mission to create a new culture of self-care and self-love in modern times.

It has been a privilege to support Susanne on the journey of publishing her insight in this book. I am proud of her for her efforts – and I know that this book will be both a guide and blessing for you in your health journey.

To your wellness and vitality!

With inspiration,

Emily Gowor

Inspirational Author & Speaker

Table of Contents

Foreword ix

Introduction 1
    You Deserve MORE! 1

Honour You 13
    Expanded Awareness - Where Are You At? 19
    Hello Beautiful - I'm Doing Me 23
    My Vision of a FULL-filled Life 29
    Transformational Goal Setting 35
    Start the Journey by Honouring You 47

Energise You 57
    The Breath of Life 61
    Love Your Sound Sleep 73
    The Essence of Life 79
    Delicious Wise Nutrition 89
    Moving With Joy 103

A Positive Attitude 117
    Choose Your Thoughts Carefully 121
    Journal Writing 125

Table of Contents

    Mindfulness Meditation 129

    Me Time 135

    Self-love - the Gift that Keeps on Giving.................. 141

Listening **145**

    The Healing Power of Listening 149

    Listen to Your Body 153

    Listen to the Rhythms of Nature 157

Touch **169**

    The Power of Touch 173

    Benefits of Hugging 177

    Meeting Your Own 'Needs' of Touch 181

    Unclothed Cognition 183

Healthy Happy Habits **187**

    Morning Ritual 191

    Evening Ritual 201

    Take Joy in Living 205

    Get Ready for Takeoff - It is Time to Thrive 209

Bibliography 213

About the Author 215

Introduction

You Deserve MORE!

I believe that the relationship you have with your body is one of the most important relationships you will ever have in life. And the truth is – it is a lifelong relationship. Other relationships will come and go, but this one will be there all the way along your Life Journey.

I meet so many women choosing to ignore the messages their bodies are sending out. They are shutting their body down, repressing it and burying their emotions, to the point of being disassociated with their own bodies and not wanting to face themselves in the mirror. They are unhappy with the way their bodies are looking, feeling, and functioning. Yes, looking in the mirror can be painful sometimes. And most of them know they can take better care of themselves. But the question is how?

Maybe this resonates with you. Maybe you feel a bit lost in the challenges of life, the struggles, and the need to be there for everyone else. Maybe you are stuck in the sadness you feel when you don't have the wellness you want. Wondering how to find your way back, back to that happy space within where you truly can say, 'I love my body' and mean it.

You and your body are travelling partners in this Life Journey so, please, start by giving your body a big HUG. Embrace the whole of You. And let us together reclaim the wellness and vibrancy you 'both' so well deserve.

Let us find those nourishing little habits that suit You. The necessary habits you deep inside know you need to be able to thrive in life. Habits you will 'vibe' with, habits you know you will keep doing because they feel right. Habits you can come back to when life stray you away from them. Yes, these habits will help keep you grounded and in a balanced state of wellness.

Please see these Healthy Habits as your wellness building blocks in life. Building blocks that work for you and that cultivate your wellness practice. Remember, sometimes it is the smallest little nuances that can make a huge difference. Yes, it's time to put yourself on top of that priority list, tune in to your needs, and start to nurture You and Your Body!

My intention with this book is to take you from where you find yourself on your Wellness Journey right now, to where you want to be. From ignorance to intentional self-love. From a state of just surviving to thriving in life. A state where you can connect to the wonderful feeling of happiness and joy within.

Introduction

This Journey starts with honouring you for all the experiences, all the 'ups and downs' you have been through in life, to looking at where you want to travel on this Wellness Journey. What does that state of balanced wellbeing and thriving in life look like for you? This is a crucial step to take. You see, if you don't know where you are going, there is a big risk of getting lost along the way. Once we have created that clarity, we will together look at different ways to re-energise, re-charge and re-new you – the important steps to take to reach your full potential and live life to its fullest.

I do believe in a broad, holistic approach to create true wellness within. For that reason, we need to find ways to nourish the whole of you - your body, mind, and spirit. Your attitude and mindset play a big part in achieving what you want in life. Both the physical and the mental aspects of you need continuous encouragement and support. Both aspects are equally important.

One of my friends once said to me, 'You can't expect beauty on the outside and be crusty on the inside.' So true! And it is also true that finding your way back to feeling vibrant and on top of the world doesn't have to be hard or take hours in the gym. A few simple strategies will get you to feeling and looking fantastic. This book will bring you there, one step at a time - one Healthy Habit at a time.

I remember when I was trekking up the very last bit to put my flag down on the mountain, over 5,700 meters above sea level in the Mount Everest region. I felt so sick and the only thought I had in my mind was 'I'm not giving up; I WILL put this flag down!' I did put it down and then ran off to throw up behind a nearby rock. Yep, altitude sickness it was and not a very nice experience either.

Life is a journey and my story about My Body and Me has been a huge part of my Life Journey. A Journey about love and acceptance, about trust and believing, about walking my talk and never giving up. Today I'm happy to say: I love myself for who I am, and I love my body for what it is. Yes, I can honestly stand in front of the mirror, naked or dressed, and say 'Hello Gorgeous' - and mean it.

Now, it was not always like that. As a teenager I hated more than loved myself and my body. I was teased and bullied for the way I looked and for being different. I developed late, was flat-chested, the female curves were 'missing', and I was the one girl missing a boyfriend. Not wanted! To top it up I apparently had a nose pointing upwards. Yep, the bullying boys in school back home in Sweden called it 'Holmenkollen,' which is the large ski jumping hill in Oslo, Norway. And I hated the feeling of my dry skin.

Whilst everybody else enjoyed playing handball, I chose gymnastics, and I was good at it. I also did well academically, and I was liked by the teachers (but that wasn't popular amongst my friends either.) So, I was a very happy camper when it was time for me

Introduction

to leave my 'pals' and move on to college and later to university, where I could build up a completely new sphere of contacts and friendship.

We are all spiritual beings, having our Human Experience here on planet Earth. Our body is the vehicle we have chosen for this Journey, so why don't we look after it and listen to the needs it has? Well, maybe you do – I certainly didn't at all to start with. I thought I was indestructible, like many other teenagers in this world. I never asked permission from my Body to do what I did. I just went ahead and did stuff and sometimes suffered badly in the process.

Our body is such an amazing vehicle. It tells us what is working and what's not – daily – and my mistake was I didn't listen. All the little sign and symptoms my body gave me, I dismissed. Sometimes it screamed loudly, and you would have thought I learned the lesson. It took me a long time and it wasn't until I started to study Oriental Medicine and the Power of Touch through a beautiful Japanese form of healing art called Shiatsu, that I started to 'wake up,' listen within, and view ME differently.

When I talk about my body and me, I don't mean just the physical me – I mean the entire Me – the physical, emotional, and spiritual Me all together. I don't think we can separate these parts. In the end we are all energy and part of the whole, so we need to take all parts into consideration. Our energy vibrates in relationship to what is within, as well as without. A sense of Balance is the key!

Think about it – what's your body made of?

- Nine systems comprise the human body including Circulatory, Digestive, Endocrine, Muscular, Nervous, Reproductive, Respiratory, Skeletal, and Urinary
- What are those made up of? Tissues and organs
- What are tissues and organs made up of? Cells
- What are cells made up of? Molecules
- What are molecules made up of? Atoms
- What are atoms made of? Subatomic particles
- What are subatomic particles made of? ENERGY!

You are – we all are – PURE ENERGY-LIGHT in its most beautiful and intelligent configuration, energy that is constantly changing beneath the surface. And you control it all with your powerful mind.

Through Shiatsu I started to understand the importance of looking after my mental, emotional, and spiritual health as a crucial part of my physical wellbeing. If you are not happy, it's hard to achieve any goal, especially health goals, and many of us go to chocolate for comfort. Chocolate for the Soul!

Yeah, some of the content in chocolate have physiological effects on the body and are linked to serotonin levels in the brain. Ninety percent of your serotonin receptors are in your gut, and serotonin is known as the 'happy neurotransmitter.' Choosing chocolate to feel happier is a choice. Maybe not the best for your health and sometimes this is the choice we make. Please, remember, in every given moment you have a CHOICE!

I made my choice – I started to invest into my own health and wellbeing and have done ever since. Shiatsu taught me that energetically we are all connected to the environment around us and to each other. Energy circulates through our body, as the river of water flows in nature, along pathways we call energy channels or meridians.

So, the studying and practising Shiatsu brought me back to nature and the wonderful healing power nature provides. This wonderful healing power of Mother Nature is referred to as Biophilia. Biophilia has become a favourite word of mine; if you think about it, when you are in nature and around other living organisms, you feel connected, you gain perspective, and life seems simpler.

This is no coincidence. Nature has a positive effect on humans' wellbeing. We thrive physically, mentally, and emotionally when we are exposed to Nature. The energy from Mother Earth helps with 'grounding,' the sun brings nourishment absorbed through the skin and helps balance your hormonal levels.

Being in the rainforest or on the beach, close to the ocean, provides us with negative ions, which is great for calming and stress reduction. All this is there for you in Nature, and the great news is – it's all for FREE, and you have unlimited access to it. It is your choice, and such a beautiful gift to give yourself - just get back to basic and back to Nature.

I grew up in Nature myself, on the countryside of Sweden, and I remember the times my mother sent me out to the veggie patch to dig up potatoes for dinner. Did I enjoy it? No, not at all, but I admit, I loved the fresh boiled potatoes served at dinner, especially the very small ones with just butter and salt on top. Yum!

I equally enjoyed the fresh, fried up mushrooms picked in the forest at autumn time and the various berries we ate. Yes, I am born a Natures Being and my parents brought me up in accordance with nature, that's for sure. I had a great start in life when it comes to food and nourishment for my cells. For that I am grateful.

My life Journey brought me to living in big cities around the world like Stockholm, New York, London, and Sydney. What I came to realise is that the further away from Nature, I found myself, the more I did seek to connect with Nature's energy in various ways. Shiatsu, Tai Chi, Yoga, and other modalities have been fabulous vehicles for me.

Today I feel I have embodied Shiatsu - it's part of my body and soul. I live Shiatsu daily and move as gracefully as I can through the different energetic movements.

Introduction

My Life Journey did finally bring me back to Nature and I now find myself living in 'paradise,' close to the beach on the magnificent Gold Coast of Australia. I chose to live according to Nature's Laws and Rhythms. I get my food from the local farmers, enjoy exercising outdoors, practising yoga, swimming in the ocean, and walking. Lately I have added Pilates to my exercise routine, and I will explain why later. I choose to wake up every morning with a smile on my face and I write in my Gratitude Journal before going to sleep. I listen to my intuition and hang around with likeminded people that lift me up. I run a business from home, built on these very principles. I believe in and I feel passionate about LIFE!

There has been a lot of self-talk over the last years, and I can honestly say I have a great relationship with my Body. We have done a couple of half marathons here on the Gold Coast, we go to the beach every morning to breathe the fresh air and walk in the sand. We take ourselves to the valley and the mountain to relax and enjoy pampering ourselves with massages and facials in between working my business from home.

Self-belief is about being the best version of you and inspiring yourself to be more. Do what you love and be real. Stop worrying about being something you are not and start being you, unapologetically. Honour yourself and chose to be around people who inspire you and love you for who you are.

Many times, have I been called 'stubborn' – another way of looking at it is being persistent and consistent…never give up on You.

I love the Chinese proverb below. It is hanging on our wall in our home, reminding me of the importance of reconnecting with myself and my inner thoughts.

If there is light in the soul,
There is beauty in the person,
If there is beauty in the person,
There will be harmony in the house,
If there is harmony in the house,
There will be order in the nation,
If there is order in the nation,
There will be peace in the world.

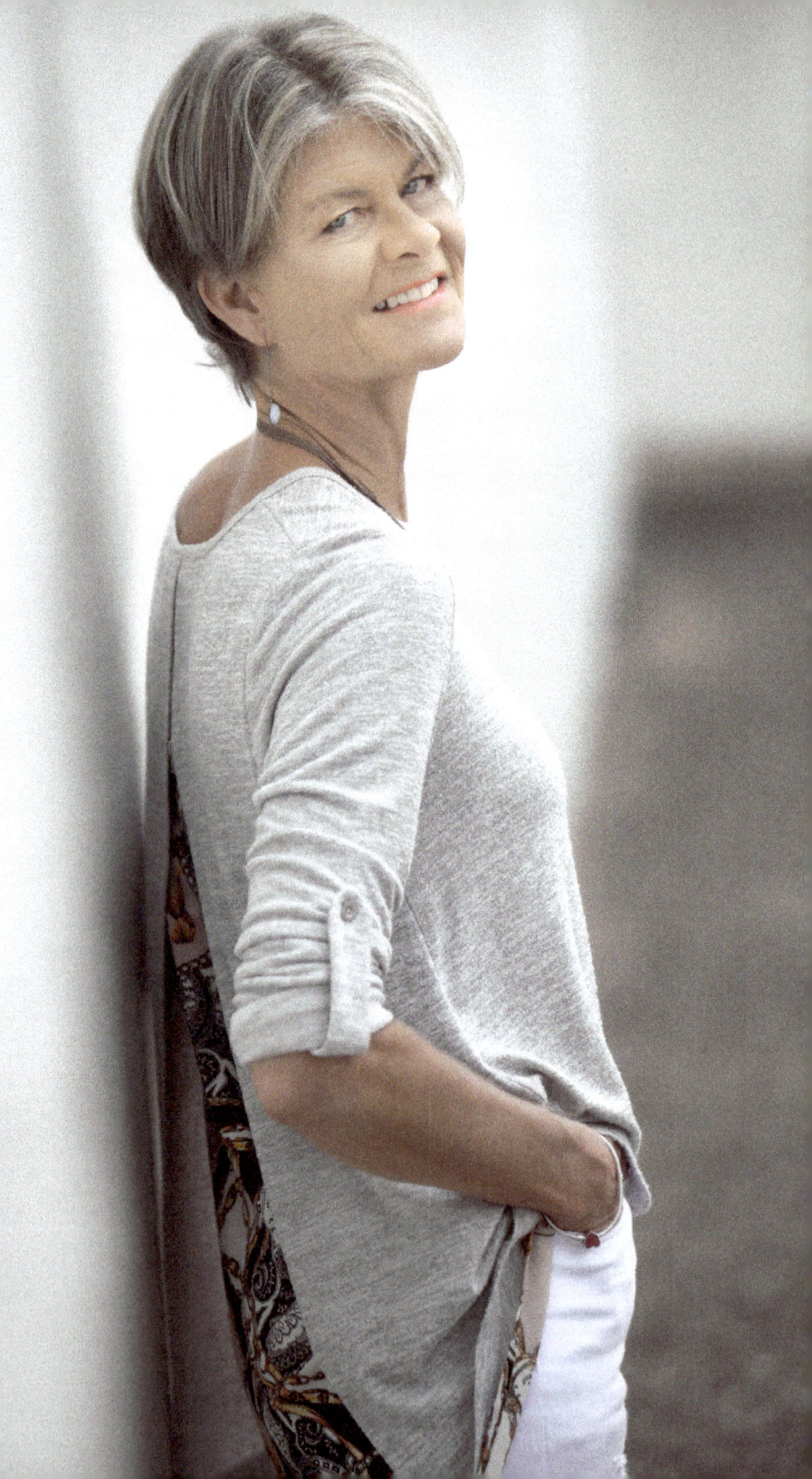

Honour You

"The quality of a person's life is in direct proportion to their commitment to excellence, regardless of their chosen field of endeavour."

Vince Lombardi

Many women I meet tend to live a very busy lifestyle. They are being pulled in one direction after the other, pushing their own needs to the back of the queue. Unfortunately, when you put yourself last it can leave you feeling drained, uninspired, and unfulfilled. You end up feeling unhappy with who you are, the stressful life you live, and unhappy with the body you live in.

The truth is, without good health, our bodies lack the energy and enthusiasm needed to do the things we love most. So, let's be clear about this, self-care is not SELFISH – it is ESSENTIAL! And you are most likely reading this because you feel it's time to take matters in your own hands and create a healthier, happier, and more vibrant You.

This is not just about looking good; it's about balance, well-being, radiant health, and beauty. The secret is simply to learn how to honour yourself with your lifestyle and the choices and commitments you have in life.

We all travel the Wellness Journey in life. Through my own Journey I have come to believe that good health goes beyond the physical. I started off in the fitness arena myself as a gymnast, dancer, PE teacher and Personal Trainer. I spent a couple of years over in New York, lived in Manhattan, and I was an exercise freak. No addictions are good for us, and I was addicted to exercise. I was teaching about fifteen classes a week, walked everywhere, and decided to run a marathon to top it up. I was on an endorphin rush 24/7, and it felt fabulous.

Yes, the body's own opiate can give you a feeling of euphoria, and I was happy with the feeling. I was probably about five kilos lighter than I am today, and I was all muscles and bones. Not a good look! The problem was, I didn't realise. As a result of this excess of exercise, my body started to scream out loudly and my back finally decided to say NO. The severe back pain my body 'gave me' stopped me completely from moving. Not a welcomed state of being in my world and 'a blessing in disguise.' My body was fed up with how I treated it – it was time for a wake-up call.

Me being me just wanted relief so I could go back and do what I loved the most – MOVE. Did you know, most people tend to move away from pain, rather than moving towards pleasure in their life? So, it was with me. What could I do to get away from this nagging back pain and get back to where I was? Now, Universe has its own ways of providing and decided to introduce me to the wonders of acupuncture, Chinese medicine, and Energy healing. This is when I started to look at health from a totally different perspective, taking in not just the physical Body, but also the Mind and the Spiritual part of myself.

Old habits die hard. Changing your habits is a process that involves several stages. Sometimes it takes a while before changes become new habits and then there are the 'roadblocks' along the way. You want habits to be simple, yet profound and easily implemented into your life. Habits that provide powerful, lasting results that sustain you, your health, and wellbeing.

Humans are habitual beings, and your life is essentially a sum of all your habits. There are four stages we go through when we change a habit, and it takes energy to get through them. And with determination, positive thinking, and a big "Why?" – you will get there one step at a time. My back pain 'helped' me to expanded awareness – stage one of the four. The four stages we need to go through are:

1. Expanded Awareness
2. Contemplation - Preparation
3. Conscious change - Action
4. Unconscious Change - Embodiment

Expanded Awareness – Where Are You At?

"We wander for distraction, but we travel for fulfilment."

Hilaire Belloc

Expanded awareness is you becoming consciously aware of the habits you want to change. This is about identifying the not so beneficial habits and choices you are living by and the impact they have had on your life. What is the negative impact it has on you and your wellbeing, your health?

We can all feel the difference between emptiness and fullness, and it is this experience that allows us to feel our way to better lifestyle choices. When you listen within and give yourself what you really want and need, your unhealthy habits – such as overeating, another piece of chocolate, that extra glass of wine, lack of exercising, in my case overexercising – cease to be a problem.

Instead of fighting against a habit that always fights back, stop yourself and ask yourself the question,

'Do I really need this right now? Is this what Me and My Body is 'hungry' for?'

Only when we have shown the light on the old habits can we begin the process of creating new ones. This is the starting point and an exciting one! This is about how you perceive yourself in reflection of your health and wellbeing – what are the positive attributes you live by and what are the ones you would like to change to create optimal health for yourself?

An Honest HEALTH check!

Your staring point involves being honest with yourself and taking 100% responsibility for all your past choices and actions. It doesn't matter where you are on your health journey; you will not make progress if you keep beating yourself up for what you did in the past. This is not about blaming and/or feeling guilty. It is simply a reality check. You will have to accept your past choices, come into the present moment, and start afresh.

To help you along the way, below are some questions to ask yourself right now – questions you want to answer honestly and truthfully. Questions that help you recognise the behaviours and beliefs that might have held you back in life. Remember, this is your check-in point, your starting point for the future You. Once you know where you are at, it becomes that much easier to set some intentions on what optimal health looks like for you. This is about creating clarity for yourself, and the exciting part is that you can make a new choice in every given moment and move forward, creating your optimal future health.

Where you are at today reflects choices, you made earlier in life. What you see in the mirror is that: a reflection of how you have been nourishing You up to this stage in your life, physically, emotionally, mentally, and spiritually. So, let's check in, with honesty and self-love in mind, and find out where You are at right now in your relationship to your body, and your overall health and wellbeing.

Health Questions for You:

1. On a scale of 1 to 10, how happy are you with your overall health and wellbeing? 10 being totally happy where I'm currently at!
2. On a scale of 1 to 10, how happy would you like to feel with your overall health and wellbeing?
3. If there is a gap between where you are at and where you want to be, why do you think there is a gap?
4. On a scale of 1 to 10, how vibrant and energetic do you feel? Your overall energy levels?
5. On a scale of 1 to 10, how happy are you with your body shape and size?
6. Do you have good nutrition practises, i.e., do you eat cleanly and avoid foods and drinks that do not agree with you?

7. On a scale of 1 to 10, on an average day, how inspired do you feel?
8. On a scale of 1 to 10, how inspired would you like to feel?
9. What is your ideal health and wellbeing outcome?
10. What would it mean to you and your life to achieve that outcome? Is it important to make a change NOW and if so, WHY?

Please write down your answers, reflect and acknowledge what is so. Acceptance is a big ask and for now, that is what might be necessary. Life teaches us many lessons and sometimes we learn the hard way. Consider those lessons as acceptances of where you are at, acceptance on why you are where you are at right now. If you can take on the belief, that all the choices you have made in your life up to now have been based on the circumstance and the tools you had at your disposal at that time, then you will accept your current situation and more easily be able to move forward. If you are ready for a change, it is time to make different and better choices. It is time to design from a place of love and compassion.

> *"Every positive change in your life begins with a clear, unequivocal decision that you are going to either do something or stop doing something."*
>
> **Brian Tracy**

Hello Beautiful – I'm Doing Me

"Success is liking yourself, liking what you do and liking how you do it!"

Maya Angelou

What does it look and feel like, the future you? Please remember that you have the power to make new choices in every given moment! New choices, new behaviours and habits moving you beyond past limitations and perceived failures. And that is all they are, your 'failures' – perceived. When you get up again and work out a better option, when you create a new path for yourself, you become a winner and a success.

As you think healthy, positive thoughts and connect with your inner wants and true power you will naturally make choices serving you and moving you towards your true potential. Health is a gift you give yourself. Healing and health come from within. It cannot be forced upon you from the outside. Listen to your body and acknowledge that you are an expert regarding your own wellbeing.

It comes back to what I said earlier: listen within! What is your heart's desire? Anything is possible and there is only one person stopping you from creating your optimal you, and that is You. Let's restore the satisfaction your life is meant to bring by starting to give yourself what you really want and need to feel inner harmony and balance. Anything that you dream and desire in your life will always manifest when your soul is in alignment with allowing it into your reality. Yes, that is what we call Divine Timing.

Contemplation - Preparation

Is it important to make a change NOW and if so, why? This was the last question I asked you to contemplate above. Contemplation and preparation are vitally important and the second stage we need to move through if we truly want to create a change of our health habits.

I believe that the key to achieving your goals in life is creating a strong reason 'WHY?'

You need to create an exciting purpose for your life and allow that to be the fuel for moving towards your future goals and intentions. A life purpose that excites and motivates you and helps you stay on track when things are not going the way you planned them to. A purpose that fills you with positive feelings when you tune into it. A purpose that helps you in those moments of doubt and despair. In those times when you are thinking the thought – Why am I doing this? Can I really do this? Nothing is going the way I want it to... That's when it is important to reconnect with your bigger WHY, your life purpose.

Your journey to reach your optimal health might not always be easy, but the truth is, it will be worth it. True happiness comes through reaching for your full potential. When you live purposefully, people will sense your energy and your excitement, and it will start to 'rub off' on others. So, not only are you transforming your life, but you will also support transforming others along the way just by being you, living on purpose.

When you are living on purpose, you have the inner knowing of where you are heading and why. You know what you need to do, and you will face obstacles and challenges with greater ease and grace. You will be able to stand up in the face of negativity and speak your own truth – speak what is so for you. You allow yourself to let go of feelings that do not longer serve, feelings of fear and self-doubt, and confidently move forward with joy and excitement in your heart.

Living on purpose creates an excitement for what is possible. We tend to connect to the bigger picture and come to realise that it is not just about us anymore, but how we can contribute to serve the good of all.

Love is the Force that moves you!

> *"It is the positive force of love that inspires you to move and gives you the desire to be, do, or have anything."*
>
> **Rhonda Byrne**

I agree with Rhonda Byrne. When I do things out of love and passion, it is very easy to stay focused to the task in hand and the result is successful. I make my choices, as we all do, and when I choose to move and do things that are in alignment with my life purpose and listen to my inner voice, my intuition, things work out well and it feels so 'right.'

I watch my son, who has great problems with focus and attention, and see him struggle to do and complete things he does not like doing. This happened very often during his school years, and it took a long time to get tasks done. On the other hand, when he occupies himself in an activity that he likes and has interest in, his focus was, and still is, fantastic! He can stay on the same task for hours, without becoming distracted, without taking breaks, and his face is 'lit up' throughout the whole process. He willingly shares his creation, and it is a pure JOY to be part of.

So, my first suggestion to you is to listen within, follow your heart, and move with love and passion in anything you choose to do. Design your future You from a place of love, compassion, and enJOYment.

The road you choose to travel will be so much easier to follow.

My Dream - My Why!

My dream is to see people on this planet be HEALTHY and HAPPY!

I love seeing healthy, happy, and joyful people. There is so much we can do to feel healthy and I'm passionate about supporting women reignite their vitality and start living their full potential. We all experience stresses in our life. When we become aware of how-to better deal with those stresses, there will be a completely new sense of calmness within. Imagine waking up feeling rested, ready for the day ahead, with the vitality and energy needed to do the things you really want to do in your life.

Through an enhanced sense of calmness within, your communication with You, will improve. Communication within the family will be easier and you will most likely find it easier to listen to others and truly hear what they have to say. With improved communication, coming from a calm space, imagine what we can create worldwide – peace on this planet. Well, that is a big dream, but why not dream Big!

My Vision of a FULL-filled Life

"NOW is the time - time to think about living your life out loud, to the fullest, unapologetically!"

Source Unknown

Clarity helps you find focus and direction. If you've ever felt lost or directionless in life, you probably know how hard it can be to make progress on anything. When you have clarity around your goals and priorities, it's easier to move towards what you want out of life.

Below is a list of questions to have you thinking about what you really want for you. Please read them and write your answers down. The more specific and clear you are in your mind of where you want to be and what you want your health and wellbeing to look and feel like, the better. Add more question to the list if you like. Allow your mind to expand and your thoughts to flow. This is about you and how you really want to live life – not according to other people's expectations. This is you, doing life on your terms.

- Where do you want to be?

- What does your optimal health look like?
- What do you want to replace the 'hunger' within with, to create fulfilment in your life?
- What body shape and size are you? What do you see when you look yourself in the mirror?
- What clothes are you wearing?
- What foods are you nourishing yourself with?
- Where do you eat? What do you enJOY drinking?
- How do you entertain and socialize?
- Who do you spend your valuable time with?
- Are you travelling the world and if so, where to?
- What do you do for relaxation? Do you pamper yourself?
- Do you spend time in Nature? If so, where?

Now, sit down, close your eyes, and see all of that clearly in front of your eyes. Visualise you, what you look like, and tune in, sense how you feel. Visualisation can be so powerful and will help bring your future you into becoming a reality - not just a dream.

The Power of a Vision Board

I enjoy creating my vision boards and they can be helpful on your health journey, transforming your life towards optimal health. Creating a sacred space that displays what you want does bring it to life.

My Vision of a FULL-filled Life

When we took the big leap of faith and decided to move from UK over to Australia, I created a vision board for myself in preparation for this huge change to occur in my life. It was a big move! I was leaving everything I had on one side of the planet and moving from the northern hemisphere to the southern hemisphere, basically as far away from 'home' as I could go. Was I nervous? You bet! Excited? Oh YES! And my vision board was a wonderful support system whenever I was in doubt about it all – such a fabulous help in keeping me on track and staying positive.

I chose a few pictures of our future living space, one being a view from a window in the house we were going to choose for ourselves. The house that was going to be our new home. It was a view overlooking the sea and some beautiful sailing boats. There was stillness in the picture and a sense of calmness around it. I could see the blue sky and a few dotted clouds. A sense of peace entered my body whenever I looked at it. The emotional connection to your vision board is vitally important!

We arrived in Sydney and spent the two first weeks house hunting. We did plenty of house viewings, but nothing felt 100% right. We did have a deadline; we were staying in a friend's place and knew we had to be out within two weeks. On the last day, I asked the agency if we could view a house we had spotted on internet before we travelled across to Australia, and she had just received the key that morning. I knew I had to view this house before making a final decision. I had a special feeling about it, and this is one time I decided to follow my intuition. I opened the door and instantly had that strong feeling, this is it! This is our house! This is where our new journey will start. Everything went quickly after that, and yes, we moved into our new home just a few days later.

Trust your intuition; it is always right!

I felt content straight away and unpacked my belongings – well, what we had then and there as most of it was to arrive a few weeks later. I looked at my vision board and that's when I realised: the view from my window was exactly as on the board. We were on the Pittwater side in Avalon, overlooking the sailing boats, and soon had quite a few nice outings in our next-door neighbors' boat.

Get Those Creative Juices Flowing

When you create a vision board and place it in a space where you see it often, you essentially end up doing short visualisation exercises throughout the day. And when you are visualising, you are emitting powerful messages out into the Universe. One of the Universal laws is the Law of Attraction. The Law of Attraction is forming your life experiences and it is doing it through your thoughts. So, whether you believe it or not, visualisation and Vision Boards work wonderfully well; so, please create yours.

My Vision of a FULL-filled Life

The purpose of your vision board is to bring whatever is on it to life. There are not any rules really on what goes on your vision board - you create your vision board on your terms in a way that 'speaks' to you. One little secret to have it work well – focus on how you want to feel. I said it before and say it again – the emotional connection to your vision board is vitally important. Choose pictures, words, and images that have you get into the feeling you want to experience in your life. Like in my example above, the view from the window had me feeling at ease and calmness within. That's exactly what I wanted in the house I chose as my home – a sense of calmness and harmony.

If you chose a picture of food you want to indulge and nourish yourself with, think about how you feel when eating it and how your body is receiving the nourishment you give it. If dancing is something that will make you happy and lifts you up, choose pictures showing that. Find inspirational quotes, notecards, or sayings you see in magazines. Do you feel excitement within when you read them? Choose those! Cut them out and put them on your vision board. Anything that inspires you to move forward with your health goals and bring the future You to life.

Place your vision board on a wall where you spend much time. You want it to be visible to you, a constant reminder, and a focus point. Whenever in doubt, whenever you feel like quitting, whenever the question 'why' comes up, look at your vision board, get into the feelings, and get back into focus.

"She silently stepped out of the race that she never wanted to be in, found her own lane, and proceeded to win."

Transformational Goal Setting

*"If you don't go after what you want,
you will never have it.
If you don't ask,
the answer is always no.
If you don't step forward,
you are always in the same place."*

Nora Roberts

Having goals and intention is the fundamental key to success. Setting goals helps us grow and expand, pushing ourselves to transform in ways we may have never imagined possible. Yes, to reach your goals takes time, diligence, the right plan, inspiration, and the right strategy, coming from a place of compassion and deep self-love. That means having integrity with your self-care and commitment to healthy practices that support and elevate your life, so you can show up fully empowered in your body.

I am a goal achiever and goal setter myself and have always been. As a young gymnast I was taught to set goals and goals were often set for me. We had our competition date; we knew our routine and our performance goals. Our coaches set a plan of action, including step-by-step training goals to achieve this. We then acted upon it, coaches, and gymnasts together as a team. We trained accordingly, with a strong intention to do our very best to achieve the goals at hand. We always moved intentionally towards them and made sure to acknowledge every little success along the way. Sometimes we hit the goals and celebrated the success and there were times when we did not reach our goals. We spent time reflecting on how we could learn from the experience and reset our target to the next time.

My father was another great goal setter and I clearly remember building our summer house. This was teamwork within the family. There were a lot of soil and rocks to move, to clear the path for a new house to be built. The three sisters shoveled dirt into the barrel and our stronger brother dumped the content of the barrel where Dad directed him to do so. Ten barrels done and we were allowed to go for a swim. Were we in full action? You bet! In the middle of a hot summer, that swim was very much wanted.

I can see clearly now…

With a clear goal in mind, the road to get there will be so much easier travelled.

A clear 'WHY?' is vitally important.
We won't be distracted by comparison
if we are captivated with purpose…

Transformational Goal Setting

If you want to succeed in achieving your optimal health, please start with setting some clear goals for yourself. Without goals you lack focus and direction, and you will much easier be distracted by 'life' happening. In the process of becoming the best version of yourself, you are going to have to sit out some tough moments.

This is when your vision board and goals come into play. Goals not only allow you to take better control of your life's direction, but they also help you stay on track and provide you with a benchmark for determining whether you are succeeding or not.

Many times, I meet women who say they set goals but never quite achieve them. A common reason for this to happen is that the goals set are not inspiring or compelling enough. Nothing great was ever achieved without enthusiasm. You are much more likely to succeed if you put your time and energy into something that excites you. When setting goals, Tony Robbins suggests we "think of a goal as a dream with a deadline!"

So, how do we set and create compelling goals? Well, it takes a bit more than just saying "I want" and expect it to happen. Goal setting is a process that starts with careful consideration of what you really want to achieve for yourself. Clearly state the goals for yourself and then put a plan of action in place that step-by-step moves you towards these goals. Following the below steps and guidelines will help you formulate achievable goals for yourself and support you in achieving the desired outcome you are wishing for.

- Set Conscious goals, goals that you clearly want and that are chosen by you and from your heart. Quiet your mind and move from your heart's desire – what is it I really, really want? Follow your intuition and listen within. Make sure your goal resonates with you and inspires you into action. You want your goals to inspire motivation! Make sure you really WANT it!

- Set Realistic goals, goals that are attainable by you. If you set a goal which you have no hope of achieving, you are not going to take action to move towards it. You will only erode your confidence. However, it is equally important to avoid setting goals that are too easy to achieve. You want to stretch yourself and feel excitement about your goals. Be a bit 'daring and disruptive' and create that inner feeling of 'I really want this to happen, and I do have the courage to go for it!'

> *"I am courageous enough to know I can accomplish great things. I am humble enough to know when to ask for help."*
>
> **Katrina Mayer**

- Set Specific goals, clearly stated and well-defined. Vague goals are unhelpful as they don't provide sufficient direction for you. The more detailed the better. The clearer the outcome you are looking for, the easier it will be to create a plan of action. Move into the feeling of having achieved the goal you are setting for yourself. What does it feel like?
- Set Time-based goals! Yep, you need to have a deadline for when you want to achieve your goals. When are you there? When will you celebrate achieving your goal? Having a clear idea of your timeline creates a sense of urgency. You will be working towards what you want more quickly.
- Set Measurable goals. Feeling happy when you look at yourself in the mirror is something you cannot measure. What is it that have you feel happy when you look into the mirror? What do you see when you look in the mirror? Is it your body shape, weight, size that has changed?
- Set Aligned goals. Goals that are in alignment with your life values that help move you in the direction you want your life and health to go. By keeping goals aligned with your bigger purpose and life values, you will develop a better sense of focus you need to get ahead and create the optimal health you want for yourself.

Grab a piece of paper and start to write down what you want to achieve to reach your optimal health and wellbeing. Go back to your list and refine it. Allow your creative juices to flow. Brainstorm a list of all the things you want to achieve, create, do, have, and experience in relation to your health and wellbeing. Give yourself time to do this, please, and allow it the time it takes.

Review your list and choose the top five goals for yourself, goals you would like to achieve within a year's time. Write them down according to the guidelines above and include why it is important for you to achieve these goals in a set timeframe. What is the outcome for you, and why is it important to move into action and create this NOW?

Now read them out loud to yourself. Do they resonate? Do they create excitement and inspiration for you enough to move into action? Do they meet the guidelines above? Do they stretch you enough? If so, great, and well done!

Next step, if possible, is to share your goals and intentions with someone. Your partner, a trusted friend, and only if this feels right for you. If not, state your goals to yourself daily. Say them out loudly, so you hear yourself. And do it with passion and joy in your voice, please.

Finally, write your goals down and put them where you clearly see them – a few different places in your home and/or your work environment. Allow them to be a constant reminder for yourself, helping you to stay on track.

In every given moment, please ask yourself the question:

- Are the actions I now choose moving me closer to the outcome I'm looking for?
- Does it serve? Does it serve me, my greater goal in life, and what I want to achieve?
- Does it serve the greater good of all?

The difference between where you are now and where you want to be is what you do!

Conscious Change - Time for ACTION

With a clear Why, with new goals and intentions in alignment with your true purpose, you are ready to move into ACTION! And to start with, I want to share with you a simple yet profound movement routine that will awaken your inner energy and truly empower you from the inside and out. A movement routine based on the traditional Chinese philosophy of energy and how it moves in a certain way in our bodies.

We are all Nature's Beings and as humans we have our own wonderful rhythms within. We are also part of Mother Earth and Nature, so for us to stay in flow and get the most out of life, to have the energy and vitality we want to have, we need to reconnect and start to move with the rhythms of Nature again.

Look at today's society and how we have surrounded ourselves with all the wonderful technologies, computers, mobile phones, electrical lights, cars – the list is long and yes, it comes with many benefits. Many of us run our businesses and life from our mobile phone, more so today than ever before. And it will continue. Unfortunately, the energy vibration from all these electric devices is detrimental for your health and disturbing to our natural energy flow. I feel we have disconnected from – divorced – Mother Nature, and I feel it is time to un-plug from time to time, to 're-marry' Mother Nature and start to thrive again.

The best way to stay healthy, according to Chinese medicine, is learning about the nature of each season and living in harmony with its spirit. When we are in tune with our bodies and how the seasons affect us, adjusting our lifestyles to coincide with the change in season is instinctual…

…However, if you're like most people, you probably don't sit around thinking about how to adjust your diet, lifestyle, thoughts, exercise, sleep, etc. to harmonise your health with the seasons.

It simply is not a part of our cultural consciousness anymore.

But, despite our lost knowledge here, learning to honour the changing needs of your body within the cycles of the seasons is a powerful way to reduce risk of common seasonal concerns of body, mind, and spirit. Slowing down and listening to your own natural rhythm can quickly reconnect you to Nature and the Universe.

Moving to the Rhythms of Nature

> *"Our biological rhythms are the symphony of the Cosmos, music embedded deep within us, to which we dance even when we can't name the tune."*
>
> **Deepak Chopra**

Nature's natural rhythms orchestrate when day turns to night, when flowers must bloom, and provide the cue for when it is time for red and brown leaves to fall from trees. As human beings, our own inner rhythm is attuned to this universal sense of timing. Guided by the rising and setting of the sun, changes in temperature, and our own internal rhythm, we have an inner knowing of when it is time to sleep, eat, or be active. While our minds and spirits might be occupied on other pursuits, our breath and our heartbeat are always there to remind us of life's pulsing rhythm that moves within and around us.

Moving to this rhythm, we know when it is time to stop working and when to rest. Pushing our body to work beyond its natural rhythm diminishes our ability to renew and recharge. A feeling much like jetlag will let us know when we've overridden our own natural rhythm. When we feel the frantic calls of all we want to accomplish driving us to move quicker than is natural for us, we may want to stop, take a few deep breaths instead. Tune in to nature moving to its own organic timing. A walk in nature can also help us reconnect to nature's natural rhythm. When we move in accordance with our natural rhythm, we can achieve all we need to do with less effort.

We may even notice that our soul moves to its own internal, natural rhythm – especially when it comes to our personal development. Comparing ourselves to others does not serve. Our best guide is to tune in, to move to our own internal timing, while keeping time with the rhythm of nature.

Energy - Ki

The concept of Ki is a fundamental concept in Eastern medical thinking, and we consider it as our 'life essence.' Ki maintains and nurtures our physical body and therefore also affects our mind and spirit. This Ki energy flows through certain pathways in our body – energy channels – called meridians. The meridians connect to our internal organs and are also named by the organs they affect. The meridians run throughout your whole body, connecting all the different body parts to one another. There are points along the meridians where the energy is flowing near the surface of the body and therefore more accessible to 'treat.' In energy medicine, this is what the practitioner is working with. An energy medicine practitioner will aim to restore balance within the meridian system to create better flow within. When there is undisturbed flow in the energy channels, there is balance in your body and mind.

Unfortunately, the flow of Ki through the meridians can be disturbed in different ways: either by external trauma, such as an injury, or internal trauma such as anxiety or stress. This is when aches and pains start to occur, and you might experience discomfort in body and/or mind.

The good news is, we can rebalance the flow ourselves. We can activate the energy channels ourselves. Like a power plant, we can transform the inner 'disturbed' energy to a higher, more useful energy source for ourselves. We can take the lower level of energy, work the meridian system, and convert it to a higher level of energy. By doing so we can generate energy into our body, into our life. How? By a simple, yet profound DoIn routine.

Start the Journey by Honouring You

"Beautiful things happen when you believe in yourself, follow your dreams, and surround yourself with positive people."

Source Unknown

The term DoIn simply refers to the 'way of exercise' and some people refer to it as self-massage. DoIn involves a combination of different techniques to activate and improve the circulation and flow of Ki throughout the whole body. These techniques include percussion, or tapping of the meridians and muscles, stretching exercises, and a wide range of breathing and movement exercises to improve your Ki flow.

Awakening and toning your meridian system ensures you are using your full potential. By practising the DoIn routine described below, you can learn to activate the meridians in about five minutes of concentrated effort. It might take a little bit longer the first time and it will get easier with practice. It is a simple and powerful way of creating a vibrant state of health for yourself. You will feel a sense of vibrancy and energy within that allows you to move and take on the day with joy and enthusiasm.

Energy on Demand! Your DoIn Routine

Preparation

Prepare yourself by gently shaking out your body. Shake your arms and hands to release any tension in your upper body. Take a deep breath in and lift your shoulders up to your ears. On the out-breath, drop them down and relax. Do this a few times, please. Gently shake out your legs and feet as well.

Place your feet shoulder-distance apart and unlock your knees. Lift up from the top of your head, straightening your back to create better energy flow and close your eyes. Take a moment to focus internally and get in touch with how you and your body feel before starting your DoIn routine. Become aware of any areas that might be in discomfort or tension. Take a few deep breaths in and out and empty your mind of disturbing or distracting thoughts.

Head, Face & Neck

Slowly open your eyes and make loose fists with your hands. Keep your wrists relaxed and gently start to tap the top of your head. Adjust the percussion pressure as needed and use your fingertips or the palm of your hand for lighter stimulation. Slowly work your way all around the head, covering the sides, front and back. Use the palm of your hand to tap the back of your head and neck area.

This exercise will wake up your brain and stimulate blood circulation, which will be beneficial for your mental focus and concentration. It will also improve the quality of your hair!

Pull your fingers through your hair a few times, stimulating the energy channels running across the top and side of your head.

Place your fingers on your forehead, apply a bit of pressure and stroke outwards from the center to the temples. Bring your fingers to your temples. Drop your elbows, relax your shoulders, and gently massage your temples, using small circular movements. This is a great way of preventing and relieving headaches.

Massage down the side of your face to the jawline. Squeeze along the jawbone, working outwards from the center. This is a very good technique for relaxation and stimulating the saliva glands at the same time.

Shoulders, Arms & Hands

Lift your shoulders up to your ears as you breathe in. Breathe out, letting your shoulders drop and relax. Repeat a few times.

Support your left elbow with your right hand and with a loose fist tap across right shoulder. Straighten your arm, open your palm, facing upwards and tap down the inside of your arm from the shoulder to the open hand. Turn your arm over and tap up the back of your arm, from the hand to the shoulder. Repeat three times.

Use your left thumb to work through your right hand. Gently massage the center of your palm, stimulating the energy point there. A wonderful and powerful way to relieve general tension and anxiety.

Squeeze and massage the joints of your fingers using your index finger and thumb. Pulling out the fingers will stimulate the starting and end points of the energy channels. A great way to release any tension in your hands and will help prevent joint discomfort.

Please take a moment and shake out both arms. Allow them to relax down the side of your body and compare the feeling in them. Your right arm probably feels lighter, more vibrant and expanded compared to the left. This just shows that there is better energy flow in the arm you just worked.

Now to repeat this sequence on the other arm, and then compare them again!

Chest, Abdomen & Lower Back

Open your chest and, using either a loose fist or open hands for comfort, tap across your chest, above and around the breasts and across your ribs. This will stimulate your lungs and enhance and strengthen your respiratory system and breathing. Children love this exercise. I often ask them to open their arms to the side of their body as the take a deep breath in. On the out breath, tap your chest and make a Ahhhhh sound! Yes, it brings a smile to your face and will help in expressing your inner thoughts and feelings. Usually a great release exercise – you feel lighter afterwards.

Proceed further down towards your abdomen and with open hands, gently tap around your abdomen in a clockwise direction – down on the left and up on the right. This follows the flow of energy and your digestion. A lovely way to help your bowels move! Do this for about a minute. Finish off working the abdomen by placing one hand on top of the other. Create circular, stroking movements around your abdomen.

Place your hands on your lower back, just below the ribcage. This is the area of your kidneys. Start to rub the area until you feel some warmth being created underneath your hands. Then proceed to gently tap the area using a loose fist. This will stimulate your Kidney energy responsible for your vitality and for warming your body.

Lean forward and place one hand on your knee. Using the back of your other hand, tap across the sacrum bone at the base of your spine. This will activate your nervous system and send energy vibrations up your spine to your brain, bringing clarity to your mental processes.

Kidney - one of our most Vital organs!

In Chinese medicine, we think about our Kidneys as the powerhouse for our body and a storage place for our reserve energy. The Kidneys store the 'essence' of who we are. This is our ancestral energy, derived from our parents and established at conception. The Kidneys are considered the 'root of life' and are responsible for many important functions in the body. Our Kidney energy:

- governs birth,
- growth,
- reproduction and development,
- and is very important for your sexual energy!

So, we want to make sure we always nurture and look after our Kidneys well, through the food we eat, through good quality sleep, through our breathing, getting enough rest, exercise, and good hydration. Want to thrive in life? Look after your Kidney energy!

On top of the kidneys sits the adrenals, closely connected to your Kidney energy. Stress and anything in excess will have a negative effect on your Kidney energy and your overall vitality. It can result in tiredness, chronic fatigue, and a general lack of zest for life.

Legs

Proceed from your sacrum to your hips and buttocks. This is usually an area where we store lots of emotions. Feelings of anger and frustration tend to get stuck in our buttocks, so please do not feel surprised if there is tension here. Moving your hips as you tap will help to release the tension and at the same time stimulate your digestive and elimination organs.

Tap down the back of your legs down to your heels, following the energy flow in the meridian system. Open your legs a bit wider and tap up the inside of your legs, all the way to the groin area. Then tap down the outside of your legs and come up the inside again. Finally tap down the front of your legs, slightly outside your thighs. Tap all the way down to your ankles and spent some time tapping your feet, using open hands. Then come up the inside of your legs again.

Finish off by coming back to your abdomen, tapping and stroking your abdomen in circular movements. Take a deep breath in, and on the out breath, let go of your shoulders and place both hands just below the navel, one hand on top of the other. This is a big energy center in Eastern medicine. We call this area the Hara or Tan Dien. Close your eyes and tune in. Breathing in and out and sensing your entire body. How do you feel now, compared to before your DoIn routine? Notice the changes, the energy flow, and the sensation within. Notice your state of being and how you feel physically and mentally afterwards.

Conclusion

Honour You by setting up this little morning routine and do it daily. It will set your foundation for creating healthier habits in your life. Allow the first thing you do in the morning to be something to 'honour you.' A gift to yourself, to acknowledge You.

Starting your day with a DoIn session will awaken your body and mind, help you feel refreshed and ready for the coming day. Repeating the routine in the evening before you go to bed will be physically and mentally relaxing and encourage a deep, peaceful sleep.

"Action expresses priorities."

Mahatma Gandhi

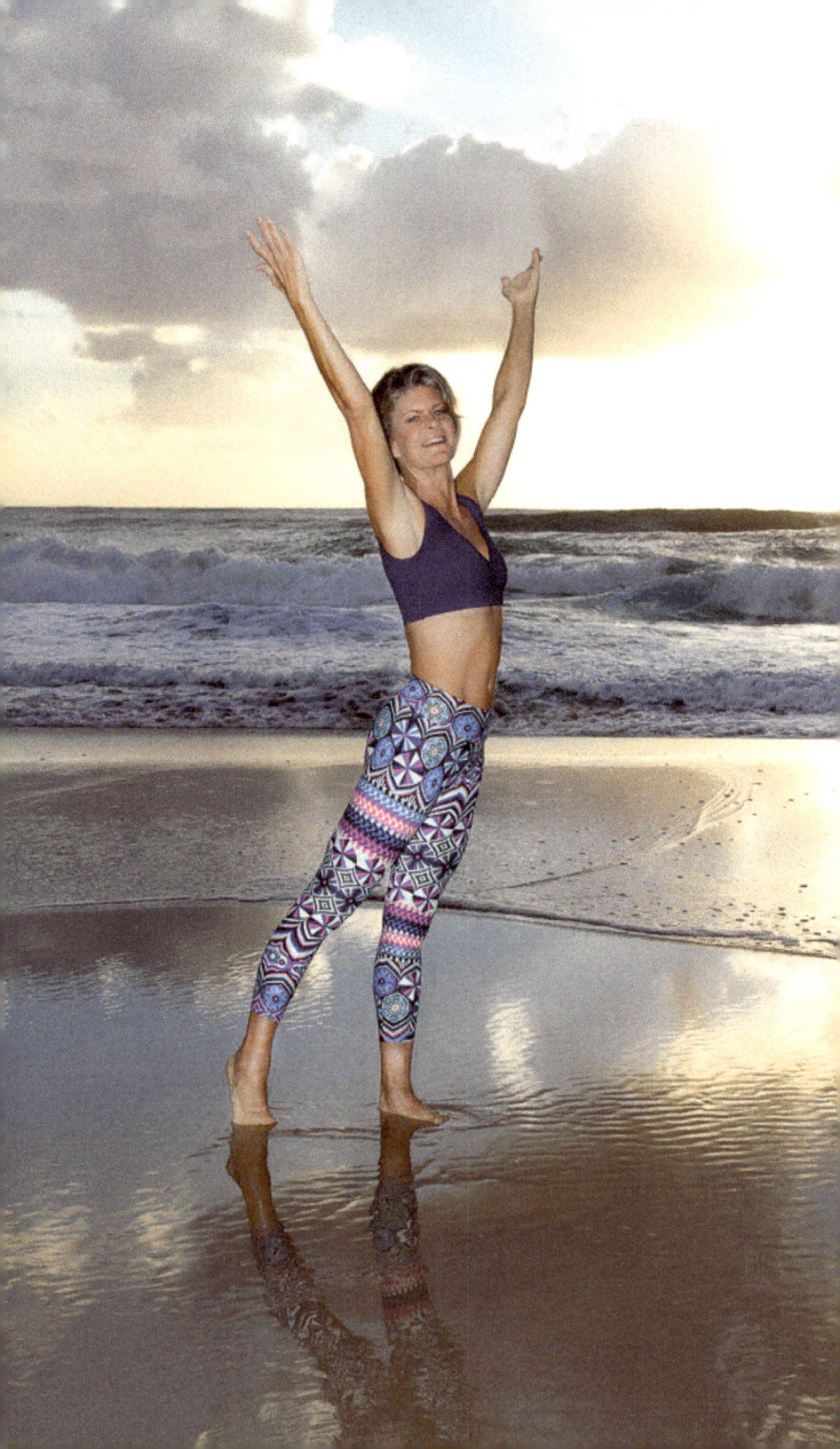

Energise You

"My mission in life is not merely to survive, but to thrive; and to do so with passion, some compassion, some humour, and some style."

Maya Angelou

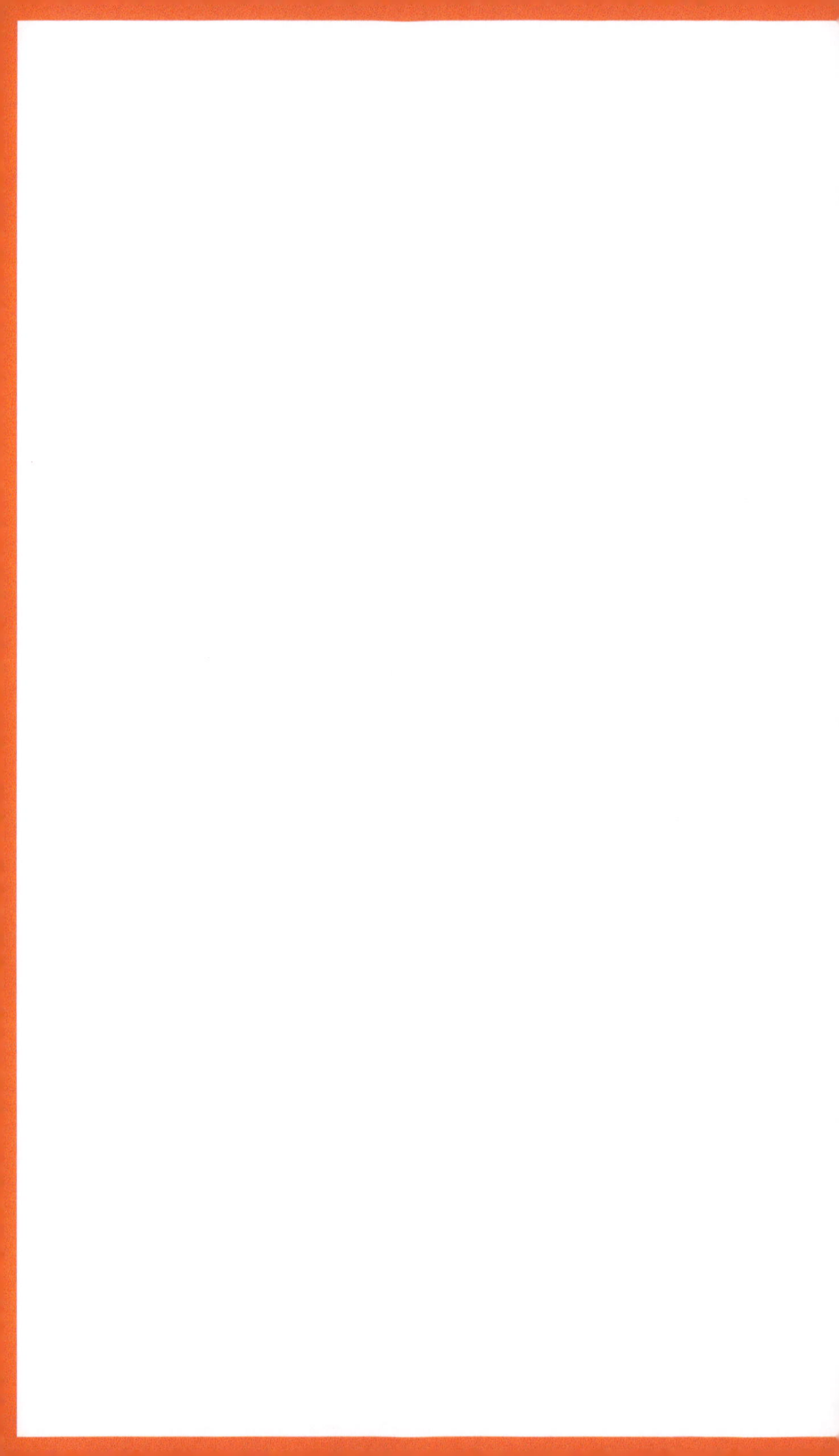

I love that quote by Maya Angelou. If you are ready, now is the time to let go of some 'bad habits' occupying your body and mind. Time to dissolve those habits that no longer serve you in exchange for some better habits. Replace them with newer, healthier habits, a new positive attitude, and a renewed connection to your true, most vibrant inner self. In this section we will look at different ways to re-energise, re-charge and re-new you, examining the steps you need and want to take to reach your full potential and live life to its fullest, with passion, lots of love, and laughter as part of it.

People are always surprised when they learn my age. I have come to a place in my life where I enjoy an abundance of energy, an active lifestyle, and living in a body I love. And I am here to tell you: you can feel this way too. It doesn't have to be hard and take hours in the gym. I have distilled it down to following a few simple steps that, whilst simple, has a profound effect.

I am about to share with you how to eat wisely, exercise enthusiastically, sleep profoundly, live in the moment, and have a passionate and curious attitude to your life.

> "The scariest moment is always just before you start."
>
> **Stephen King**

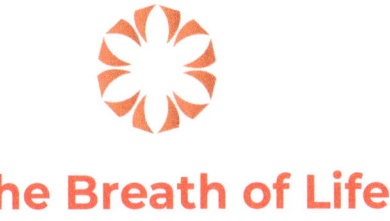

The Breath of Life

"Breathe. Let go. And remind yourself that this very moment is the only one you know you have for sure."

Oprah Winfrey

The first thing we do as newborns is take a nice, deep breath of air into our body. And when we are ready to leave this space and move on, when we die, we passively breathe out – the breath of life leaves us.

Think about it; you can live for weeks without food, days without water, but how long without air? Not very long.

Yes, you are breathing right now – automatically. The air flows in and out through your nose without you having to think about it. Unless there is a health issue you are dealing with, breathing is an automatic process, and it has its own rhythm in your body. It happens about 25,000 times a day – yes, that is how many breaths you take daily.

Yet, my question to you is – are you really breathing? Are you bringing that energy from the air, through the lungs all the way down into the whole of your body? Are you giving your whole body the possibility and opportunity to utilise the powerful energy from the air?

I was trekking in Nepal a few years ago with my husband. We did a 16-day trek in the Mount Everest region and our final goal and destination was a place called Kalapathar, located over 5,700 metres above sea level. A lot of planning went into the whole trip, and we were very excited about the adventure. The first part of the trek was wonderful and quite easy. We were well prepared physically and closely followed the guidelines regarding how fast to move up the mountain. Yes, we had a plan to reach our end destination in the time available.

As we reached higher and higher altitudes during the trek, the lack of oxygen and the effect of not getting enough of it became very clear to me. It was difficult to breathe, and it affected my strength, vitality, and the speed at which I walked. Amazing how the body had to adapt! I clearly remember that last day, reaching the top and the slow pace we all walked in. Placing one foot in front of the other, slowly moving up the mountain, getting to where we wanted to go. Breathing deeply with every step, trying to get as much as possible out of every breath I took and finally reaching our goal. It included a lot of will power, not giving up, and a great deal of determination and patience on my part. I did suffer altitude sickness, but I did reach my goal. It was a wonderful experience to finally put that flag down, and for me, such a great example of the importance of oxygen for my health and wellbeing. A learning experience for sure!

Oxygen as a Source of Energy

In Chinese medicine, we serve our body with energy from two major sources: the food we eat and the air we breathe. The food and air we take in is internally transformed into a more usable energy form in your body – an energy form you can use for your activities and processes throughout the day.

Air enters the body via your lungs and through your breath you bring oxygen to your internal environment. Breathing then becomes a very important part of our vitality. Our lungs are the organ connection here, so enhancing and strengthening our lungs and our breath is the focus we want to give.

There are three main compartments to the lungs and unfortunately many of us practice shallow breathing, where the breath just reaches into the upper lobes of the lungs. This will have a direct effect on things like our memory, our energy and vitality as well as our immune system, as we only take in a small amount of air and the oxygen contained in that small amount of air will have to nourish every single cell in our body.

Deep Breathing

The best way to strengthen our lungs is to breathe deeply. It sounds so simple and yet most of us don't breathe deeply at all. When you breathe deeply and with intention you are flooding your cells and your brain with much-needed oxygen that is vital to all the different processes within your body. Yep – your cells BREATHE. The air does not just come into your lungs. The exchange of oxygen is happening in very small parts of your lungs called the alveoli and is then taken to every single cell in your body via your circulation system. Every cell in your body inhales the oxygen and exhales the carbon dioxide – a process called respiration.

I see it as an exchange with the external environment. Letting go of toxins and what is no longer needed. Allowing new fresh energy to enter through the lungs. This can include letting go of thoughts and beliefs you no longer want to hang on to or letting go of negativity in your life – any negative thoughts you might have that are stopping you from moving forward to where you want to go and what you want to create. You can let go of beliefs that no longer serve your future health and wellbeing. Negative experiences are metabolised differently than positive experiences. If you overload the system with negative input, it goes out of balance. Expel them through your out-breath and create space for new, more beneficial thoughts and belief patterns to enter.

Now, with your in-breath, bring in some positivity and light instead. Thoughts that feed you on every level of you being. Supporting you to be the healthy, happy you that you want to be. If you substitute positive inputs instead, these also get metabolised into your overall wellbeing, energy level, and health.

Positive experiences that make you feel lighter physically and emotionally, from the freshest organic foods to laughter, to the beauty of Mother Nature. Positive input strengthens you on every level, making it much easier to rid your system of toxins.

I was teaching a Shiatsu workshop in Italy and practising some of my favourite breathing exercises with the students. I got to learn the Italian word for breathing out and breathing in: espirare (breathing out) and inspirare (breathing in). 'Inspirare,' very close to the English word 'inspire.' With every breath you take, you inspire your body and mind. Such a nice way of thinking of our breath - see your own in-breath as inspiration for You and your body! What do you breathe in?

How to practice Deep Breathing

To support deep breathing, consider your posture and how you hold yourself. A collapsed chest does not allow for deep breathing to happen. Lift up from the top of your head and open your chest, without forcing it. Allow your eyes to look ahead of you, rather than glancing down to the floor. Relax your shoulders and let your arms hang relaxed along the side of your body. Put a hand on your chest and a hand on your belly and breathe. To start with, just check where your breath stops and become aware of your breathing. Does it feel easy to breathe? Is it a nice flow? Do you ever feel out of breath?

Then take a deeper breath in to your lungs, allow the breath to travel all the way down to your belly and fill up that space, feeling your belly expanding. Now you are practicing deep breathing. Now you are feeding your body the energy from the air it needs to have.

The best time of the day to practice some breathing exercises is first thing in the morning. In the Eastern world, people will be out around four to five a.m. to practice their Tai Chi and Chi Gong movements, as well as airing their pets – dogs and birds in cages come out to breathe with them.

This is the optimal time during the day to better your lung energy and feed your body vitality through your lungs. This is when the air is fresh; this is Lung time, the time of the day when your Lung energy is in action and moving.

If you have the opportunity, create space and time in the morning to go for a short walk and focus on your breathing. Step outside in the garden and do some opening chest exercises. Smell, hear, and feel nature around you and allow yourself to be filled with what Mother Nature has to offer. Or open your bedroom window and take in a few deep breaths. Find your space and your time to breathe and bring focus into it. I tend to go for a walk on the beach every morning, and I realise not everyone can do this, but please find your way. The calming effect it has on you is well worth the effort.

Whenever you feel stressed and uptight, nervous, excited or in a rush – please, take a moment to stop! Take a few deep breaths there and then, wherever you are, to calm the nervous system and focus your breath and energy in the center of yourself. All the way down to your feet. Feel grounded and supported by Mother Nature and then move forward with your actions. Your Body will thank you for it!

Your Skin – an Extension of Your Lungs

We also 'breathe' through our skin, the largest organ of the body. If you think about it, this is another exchange with the external environment. Whatever you put on your skin, from the water you shower and swim in, to the moisturiser and body lotions you use to smooth and hydrate your skin from the outside – all of this gets absorbed through the skin into your body. When too hot, you sweat and let go of toxins.

Your skin acts as a protective barrier between the outside and the inside of your body. So, what you put on your skin matters. We want the inside of our body to be alkaline. Why? In an alkaline environment, illness doesn't thrive. The pH of the skin on the other hand is acidic. To look after the health of your skin and the protective layer of yourself, please make sure you use skin products that are pH balanced for your skin, i.e. acidic. When using alkaline products on your skin, you will damage the protective barrier and allow toxins to enter your body through your skin. Wrong pH balanced skincare can also cause other problems, like eczema and irritability of the skin.

As a teenager I had very dry skin and I used lots of hydrating lotion to soften it up. Drinking good quality water and plenty of it made a huge difference. When looking at skin care products for myself, I now also make sure they have hydrating ingredients. This is important when it comes to both body moisturisers as well as facial products.

Hyaluronic acid is a sugar that is naturally produced by your body. It is found in our skin and is responsible for the skin's plumpness and volume. It acts a bit like a sponge and helps retain moisture in your body. Hyaluronic acid can draw in moisture and increase the hydration content in the epidermis so that it looks and feels soft, supple, and radiant.

Essential for maintaining the skin's moisture balance, hyaluronic acid also helps smooth the texture of your skin. Unfortunately, the skin's natural production of hyaluronic acid declines as we age, which is why it is important to supplement the skin with skincare products that contains this very important ingredient.

In Chinese Medicine our Lungs are connected to our Large Intestine. Another organ we use for letting go of stuff. What you don't manage to let go of through your digestive system and your bowels, sometimes comes out through your skin instead. Excess can show up as skin eruptions, pimples, and boils.

The outside reflects your inside – yes, the condition of your skin reflects your internal environment. You can't be crusty on the inside and expect beauty on the outside. This is your body communicating with you and letting you know what is going on with you, on the inside. Be observant and act accordingly!

Start to look after your skin by doing skin cleansing. Not only cleaning of you face, but your entire body. The truth is, during sleep your body is hard at work. One thing your body is busy doing when you are asleep is detoxing your systems and your organs.

When you wake up in the morning your body is covered by lots of dead skin cells - yep, plenty of dead skin cells in your bed as well. So, if you don't shake out your sheets every morning, you go to sleep on your 'leftovers'. A scary thought and it is true. An easy and quick way to help you rid yourself of these dead skin cells is practising some skin brushing.

Dry skin brushing is excellent for exfoliating rough, dry skin. It unclogs pores and helps detoxify your skin by increasing blood circulation and promoting lymph flow/drainage. Dry brushing can be done daily over the whole body, preferably in the morning before you go into the shower. Please start with a gentle brush and soft pressure. How you touch and work your skin matters. Come from a point of love and give your body attention when doing your skin brushing. You can then work up to a firmer brush and more firm pressure over time if you like. Below are some guidelines to follow:

1. Start at your feet and move up your body
2. Use wide, circular, clockwise movements when you brush your skin
3. Use a light pressure in areas where your skin is thin and soft. You can use firm pressure on thicker skin, like the soles of your feet. Be conscious of what you do and listen to your body's needs
4. Brush your arms after you brushed your feet, legs, and mid body areas.

Dry brushing has numerous proven benefits, from increasing circulation, as already mentioned, to improving the skin's appearance by stimulating cell renewal. The theory behind brushing toward the heart is that by making long, sweeping strokes in the direction of the heart, you are working with the body's lymph flow.

This is great in promoting better lymphatic drainage. By improving lymphatic drainage your skin appears more beautiful. Moving the lymph helps reduce oxidative stress caused by free radicals by removing the toxins and other harmful substances. Reducing fluid retention means the skin will appear less puffy and blotchy.

It doesn't stop there – a more efficient lymphatic system can reduce the effects of delayed onset muscle soreness and decrease swelling, muscular fatigue, weakness, and pain! Voila – add skin brushing to your daily habits and improve your future health and wellbeing. Yes, your body will thank you for it.

Please remember to look after your face in the same nourishing way. A good skin care routine starts with cleansing. Choose a product that works with the quality of your skin type. There are some lovely devices for cleaning your face and many cleansing products to choose between. Do your research and think about the above – pH balanced skin care that includes ingredients that helps with hydration. Avoid brushes as they might damage your healthy skin cells. You want to remove the unhealthy skin cells and protect the healthy ones.

Use skincare that allows your skin to breathe. You do not want to clog up your pores with your skincare.

Remember, you breathe through your skin, and keeping a healthy skin care routine will benefit your overall health and wellbeing. And allow you to glow!

> *"Life is not measured by the breaths we take, but by the moments that take our breath away."*
>
> **Maya Angelou**

Love Your Sound Sleep

"Sleep is an investment in the energy you need to be effective tomorrow."

Tom Rath

For me, sleep is the foundation for our health and wellbeing. Why, may you ask? During sleep you give your body the chance to rejuvenate and recharge your batteries. Yes, all your little millions of cells get re-vitalised when you are in deep sleep. You build up your immune system and give your body the opportunity to perform repair work. Without sleep you would not survive! So, let's make sleep your best friend.

Getting enough quality sleep every night is one of the most fundamental aspects for human health, yet about 40% of adults suffer from insomnia. To have the health and vitality you want, it is important to make sleep a priority. According to the National Sleep Foundation, adults need between seven to nine hours of sleep every night. But it isn't enough to look at the quantity of sleep, the quality of sleep is even more important to consider.

Many of the women I work with suffer from sleep deprivation, having them lacking in vitality, low libido, irritability, and low energy levels. Ongoing, continuous sleep deprivation can over time lead to weight gain, high blood pressure, stroke, heart diseases and many other serious problems.

Sleep and wellbeing go together and getting a good night's sleep is just as important to your overall health as eating well and exercising regularly. You need that good quality sleep to revitalise, recharge your batteries, and rebuild any 'damages' within. Think of your body like a factory. As you drift off to sleep, your body begins its night-shift work. Yes, there is a lot of work going on within your body as you lay down to rest:

- healing of damaged cells and tissues
- deep quality sleep builds up and boosts your immune system
- recharging the 'energy batteries' and recovering from the day's activities
- recharging your heart and cardiovascular system for the next day
- detoxification and getting rid of what's not needed

What happens if we don't get enough sleep?

If your body doesn't get a chance to properly recharge during the night (by cycling through the two phases of sleep, REM and non-REM), you are setting yourself up for disadvantage the next day. You might find yourself:

- feeling drowsy or moody – haven't we all experienced this one…?!
- struggling to stay focused, remembering things, or making decisions
- craving coffee, tea, or other stimulants and even more unhealthy foods, which could cause weight gain. How about some chocolate!!!

One night of bad sleep every now and then is ok. Your body can probably deal with that, but if this continues to happen night after night, you can just imagine the strain it would place on your nervous system, your body, and overall health and wellbeing.

Everything in life has its own rhythm and cycles, and your body cycles through two recurring phases of sleep: REM (rapid eye movement) and NREM (non-REM or non-rapid eye movement). Both these phases are important and relate to different functions in your body. For example, a hormone that is essential for growth and development is only released in the last stage of NREM sleep.

If the REM and NREM cycles are interrupted multiple times throughout the night, either due to snoring, difficulties breathing or waking up frequently throughout the night, then we miss out on some vital body processes, which can affect our health and well-being not only the next day, but on a long-term basis as well.

Profound SLEEP

Preparation is a great start...!

What I mean by this is to prepare yourself, your body and mind, as well as your sleep environment for the activity at hand: deep, revitalising sleep! The environment you sleep in is vitally important if you want to have a good night's sleep. Some hints for you:

- Spend some time in natural light throughout the day. This helps promote melatonin production in your body. Melatonin is a hormone that allows you to 'know' when to sleep and when to wake up.
- Complete your exercise earlier in the day, not just before bedtime. Gentle yoga stretches are better. You are preparing your body for stillness!
- Eat and drink a few hours before bedtime and avoid stimulating food, spices, and drinks. I enjoy herbal teas at night, teas that support relaxation of body and mind.
- Aim to go to bed at the same time every night and wake up at the same time every morning. Create this rhythm for yourself and your body and you will soon find that you naturally are drawn to bed when that time is coming, and you might even find yourself waking up without your alarm in the morning.

- Please remember, your bedroom has two purposes only: rest and intimacy!
- Look after your sleep environment. Declutter, so you have space to 'breathe.' In my bed, there is only me and my husband, no 'extra' stuff that might irritate me. My bedside table will have my Gratitude Journal, a photo, and a glass of water on it – and my night light. I don't have too much on the walls in my bedroom. Just a few pictures enhancing my unconscious to be in the right energy space for sleep to happen.
- Make sure you have plenty of fresh air - open windows. Keep your bedroom cool, quiet, and dark.
- Remove all electrical devises, your mobile phone - you really want to unplug from the electromagnetic smog we tend to live in throughout the day. If you need an alarm clock to wake up, please invest in a simple battery drive one.
- Please use your bed only for sleep (and intimacy!). This is not the space for watching television, studying, eating, or working. You want your body and brain to associate your bed with rest and relaxation. Make sure it is comfortable, giving you the support and warmth needed to feel relaxed when lying down. Set it up for deep quality sleep.

- Go to bed with an 'empty mind' – let go of the stresses and happenings during the day AND be grateful for all the positive things you had happen throughout the day.

Sleep also affects the bodies growth hormones, melatonin, cortisol, leptin, and ghrelin (this hormone helps regulate food intake, bodyweight, and your glucose balance). By getting enough sleep you are not only allowing the body rest but also balancing your hormones. Most of us women know about that one. Balanced hormones – happier mood. Make sleep your best friend.

In Chinese medicine, the sleep cycle is also part of our shen, spiritual activities. Shen in Chinese medicine refers to thought, state of consciousness, and mental functions that keep the mind sharp and alert. It is the highest authority of the physical body that orders it to rest or work. Shen 'hides' in the organs at night for recharging and comes out during daytime to exert its duties. Sometimes when she is too excited – for example during emotional conflict – sleep problems occur.

The Essence of Life

> *"You are not sick - You are thirsty. Don't treat thirst with medication."*
>
> **Dr. Batmanjhilidj**

Water! A key element in looking after your energy powerhouse, your Kidneys!

Enough of it, and yes, in 'lagom' amounts! (Lagom is a Swedish word for not too much, not too little... just the right amount!) Water: we turn on the tap and there it is. Reliable, plentiful, and inexhaustible. We take it for granted, and we should not really, because without it we would not survive for more than a few days. Water is essential to life!

We all know this, and you might also know the adverse effects on your health when you don't get enough of it. Yet, it is well recognised that a large proportion of the population is clinically dehydrated. Sports scientist Dr. Michael Colgin estimates that more than 90% of our population over the age of 25 is chronically dehydrated. The world-famous Dr Batmanjhilidj considers dehydration to be at the root of nearly all disease including cardiovascular and cancers.

Drinking plenty of water is such a key ingredient to our health and vitality. Staying well hydrated is vital for everything you do in life really – exercising, maintaining your energy levels; and it is a key element for slimming down and toning up.

You Really Are a Body of Water

Water circulates through our body, just as it travels through the earth, cleansing, invigorating, giving life, and sustaining energy. Water is the basis of all life and that includes our body.

- Your muscles that move your body are 75% water.
- Your blood that transports nutrients are 82% water.
- Your lungs that provide your oxygen are 90% water.
- Your bones are 25% water.
- It even shapes your thoughts, as 76% of our brain, the control centre of your body, is water!

You could say – you are what you drink. Not what you eat.

I am passionate about supporting people to great hydration, and there is a very good reason for this. I was so badly dehydrated once in my life I passed kidney stones! Painful and not something I wish upon anyone, and it does happen and for me as a direct result of dehydration. Some women who have experienced kidney stones as well as childbirth, tell me the pain is equal or worse. My reflection to that: I'd rather end up with a beautiful baby in my arms, rather than some small little kidney stones I had to pass to get rid of the pain...

How did I manage to create this for myself?

Well, we were travelling to Israel to teach a Shiatsu workshop and had decided to stay at the airport hotel, as we needed to be there extremely early in the morning hours to check in. We arrived and checked in to the hotel, had a nice evening meal and a wonderful sleep in the air-conditioned room. Not good for your hydration levels, air condition!

All was good and we got up early to do what we needed to do. This is when it happened. My back started to ache, and I knew it was either something to do with my reproductive system, or my kidneys. The intensity of the pain increased but if I could move, stretch, and use the trolley, I could avoid the pain and I was ok.

This worked until I strapped myself into the seat on the aircraft – the pain got so bad I fainted from it. I woke up to the air stewardess asking me if I was alright. Of course, I said 'Yes, I'm fine!' I was not going to get off the plane after all those hours of getting there, and knowing it was a packed plane and everyone else just wanted to get going and reach their destination. I was staying where I was! Very determined!

Unfortunately, I managed to faint again, and the pilot decided he did not want to fly with me on board. A bit dramatic with the ambulance rolling up to the runway, me trying to get off the plane without anyone 'seeing' me. I very much disliked being the nuisance for everyone else's delay – funny how we think of others rather than ourselves in these kinds of situations. Plus, they had to find our luggage and take it all out of the plane, which caused further delay for everyone. Off to the hospital we went, and yes – kidney stones it was.

Now, did I learn from the experience? Not really, and being a natural health therapist, I knew the importance of drinking enough water already. Having said that, I did not drink enough. I passed kidney stones twice more following this incident. My excuse: water did not really 'agree' with me, and I thought herbal teas and other drinks were hydrating me enough. Not true. We need pure, good quality water to hydrate.

Today, having changed my habits, drinking good quality water that my body absorbs better, and enough of it daily, I am happy to say my internal, cellular hydration is brilliant. My skin feels fabulous and soft to the touch and my energy levels are so much more balanced.

Dehydrated - What Does it Look Like?

If you are thirsty, it is already too late - it means your cells are already dehydrated. A dry mouth should be regarded as the last outward sign of dehydration. That's because thirst does not develop until body fluids are depleted well below levels required for optimal functioning. The effects of even mild dehydration include tiredness, lack of focus and concentration, decreased coordination, dry skin, decreased urine output, dry mouth and nose, blood pressure changes and impairment of judgment.

Stress, headache, back pain, allergies, asthma, high blood pressure and many degenerative health problems can be the result of dehydration. Here is another interesting one for you - one of the first signs of dehydration is hunger! Next time you are feeling peckish, try drinking a big glass of water and feel the hunger go away.

A good way of checking your hydration level is keeping a check on your urine:

- A well hydrated body produces clear, colourless urine.
- A slightly dehydrated body produces yellow urine.
- A severely dehydrated body produces orange or dark-coloured urine.

How Much H2O and When?

Simply improving hydration can help increase the body's ability to transport nutrients to cells and to flush unwanted toxins out of the system. When my clients ask for a 'detox' regime, the first thing I recommend is to increase their water intake. It is best to replace fluid after your body excretes it. As water loss happens during sleep, a good start to the day is to drink a couple of glasses before breakfast. Then evenly consume water throughout the day.

Morning is when you are most full of toxins and dehydrated. Yes, when at rest your body is hard at work and detoxification is one of the important processes that is happening when you are sleeping. Some of those toxins are collected in your mouth. Hence that not so good taste in your mouth and a layer on your tongue when you wake up. So, if you grab that big glass of water straight away upon waking up - what are you doing? You are swallowing down those toxins your body just rid itself of and gulping them back down into your system again.

So, before reaching for that big glass of water, please rinse your mouth and/or brush your teeth. Then drink a big glass of fresh water and enjoy it. If you add a bit of freshly squeezed lemon to it, brilliant! That will help your internal environment become alkaline. Illness does not thrive in an alkaline environment, so having a glass of lemon water first thing is working preventative with your future health and wellbeing. To top it up, this water in the morning really gets the blood flowing.

To support the digestive process, drink water prior to and after your meals. The stomach depends on water to help digest food, and lack of water makes it harder for nutrients to be broken down and used as energy. The liver, which dictates where all nutrients go, also needs water to help convert stored fat into usable energy. If you are dehydrated, the kidneys turn to the liver for backup, diminishing the liver's ability to metabolise stored fat. The resulting reduced blood volume will interfere with your body's ability to remove toxins and supply your cells with adequate nutrients.

Following that first glass of water, drink another glass before breakfast and then another glass before starting your daily activities. This way you will have started your day with drinking close to a litre of water already. The recommended intake of water for an adult, is one litre per 25 kg of body weight. This results in 2 - 3 litres per day for most women. I suggest you check in with yourself and mark down how much water you drink daily. Then be 'daring' and take on the challenge below.

Water Challenge:

Following the first three glasses of water as per above, drink one big glass of water on the hour every hour for the rest of your day! Always keep a bottle of water with you.

- If exercising, you need more.
- If in air-conditioned space, you need more.
- If out in the sun and sweating, you need more.
- If sitting in front of a computer, you need more.

This might be a challenge for you as it was for me to start with. Now I am persistent and consistent in my water intake. It has become a healthy habit and my body is so much happier.

Without water, or with too much of it, our optimal hydration levels get out of balance and our health and normal body functions suffer. Our body is amazing! It attempts to keep a water balance internally and when the balance is out, it sends us signals. We feel the need to urinate when there is an overflow, and we feel thirsty when there is a need of water. If you don't drink water, it can lead to kidney stones, urinary tract infections, migraines, constipation, stress, and depression – the list is long.

Make drinking water a habit and you will also enJOY these wonderful benefits:

- Weight loss, helps flushing out by-products of fat and other unwanted toxins
- Temperature control - helps cool down your body when overheating through producing sweat
- Muscle efficiency - being well hydrated is essential for keeping those muscles strong, lubricated, and energised. Why? Because water aids transport of oxygen to your muscles so they are prepared when exerted.
- Skin quality; help keep your skin moist, supple, and elastic

- Balancing mood, as it helps brain function
- Memory - oh yes, proper hydration will improve the blood flow and oxygen flow to your brain, strengthening cognitive function and memory!
- Immune system and PAIN - helps fighting off illnesses, improving lymph fluid within the immune system and preventing headaches, joint pain, muscle weakness, fatigue, and light headedness.

Make hydration a habit!

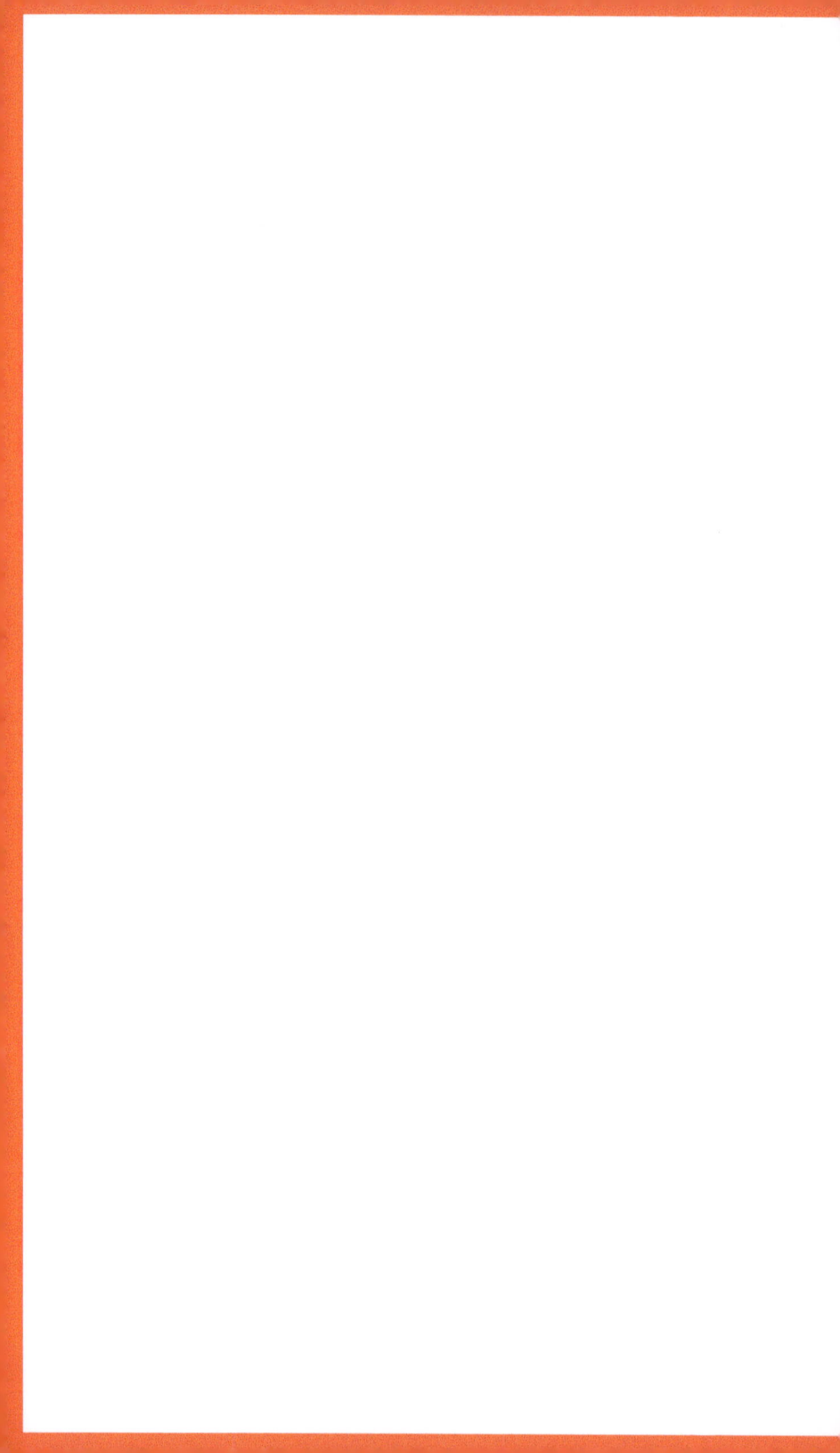

Delicious Wise Nutrition
"Food - nourishment for Body & Soul"

Let's look at the role food plays for your vitality and health. A balanced and well-rounded diet includes protein, carbohydrates, and fats. Each meal you consume should have elements of each of these. How much and size of your portions depends on your level of activity, gender, and your personal goals. As a rule of thumb, have most of your carbohydrates in the morning and reduce the amount per meal as the day progresses.

Carbohydrates

Carbohydrates provide the body with glucose, which is converted to energy used to support bodily functions and physical activity. Carbs are essential for energy, building lean muscles and normal body function. They help fuel your brain, kidneys, heart muscles and your central nervous system. Unfortunately, many of us over consume carbs and consume them at the 'wrong' time of the day.

Protein

Every cell in the human body contains protein. You need protein in your diet to help your body repair cells and make new ones. Yes, protein repairs muscle tissue and helps promote muscle growth to boost your metabolism. Protein is great for keeping you satisfied and helps reduce those food craving you might have – cravings of carbs, for example.

Unlike carbohydrates and fats our body cannot store protein. If the protein you consume isn't used, your body will rid itself of it. Hence, it is important to include protein in all your meals.

Fats

Good fats are essential for balancing your blood sugar levels and curbing unwanted cravings. Fats are your body's basic building blocks. Transporting important vitamins throughout the body, such as A, D, E, and K. These vitamins can't be absorbed in your intestine without fat. Why? They are fat-soluble, which means they can only be absorbed with the help of fats. And you want them in your body - to feed a nice sharp brain, big heart, and eagle eyes. I love my avocados! You also find good fats in olive oil, nuts, and eggs.

Food as Nourishment

I grew up on the countryside of Sweden, a country with four very distinct seasons, and I learned to live according to the seasons when it came to nourishing and feeding myself. We had a big garden and vegetable patch. My siblings and I had our own little patch to oversee. Did I enjoy the work included? Mostly not, but today I'm very grateful for the learning my parents provided.

I was taught how to fertilize the soil, plant the seeds, look after the little seedlings, and pull out the weeds. Nourish the plants and follow their growth to time of harvesting. What I enjoyed the most was that last bit – harvesting and eating them!

Yes, pulling up that little carrot from my own veggie patch, wiping it clean on the grass, and then munching away on the sweetness of it. That was YUM and such a nice reward for me. To be able to go into the garden and pick berries for dessert, or just because I felt like it – such wonderful memories!

During the autumn, we harvested whatever was growing in the garden and filled the food cellar with potatoes, carrots, and preserved things in different sized jars. Pickled beetroot and cucumber, beans, and radishes. Some things went into the freezer.

We went to the forest to pick the autumn mushrooms and berries. Mushrooms were dried, berries were made into compotes and cordial, plums were preserved in jars. It was a pleasure to see the food cellar being filled in preparation to sustain us during the winter season when nothing is growing. Not much grows in snow! Mother Nature goes into hibernation and so do many of nature's animals.

Since my childhood I have been through different food regimes. I have been vegetarian, vegan, and tried a few different types of diets. What I have come to realise is, that if you carefully learn to listen to what your body needs and thrives on, you will find the right foods that work for you.

The food philosophy I like the most and align myself with is macrobiotics. In macrobiotics we learn to eat what is in season and what grows in our local environment. Why, might you ask? Because what grows in your neighbourhood and what's in season has the most energy to offer you and your body. This resonates with me as I want to nourish my body with food that gives me energy and vitality.

Back to Basics

If we nourish ourselves with food and look at the outcome being energy, please start eating 'Real Food' and foods that are in season. What do I mean with that? Go back to eat basic, take yourself to the Farmer's Market. Choose quality, rather than quantity. Eat organic when possible. Look at the ingredients list, rather than the calories in the food you buy. Avoid sugar, preservatives and any colouring. This is just chemicals and will not do you and your body any good – it will create toxins and make your body work harder to clean up again.

Food is nourishment and has come to stand for many other things - fulfilment of other needs. 'We are what we eat' is a very common saying and I bet you have heard it a few times. Is it true though? It was for me until I met someone telling me it was not! It does not matter how much great food you put into your mouth, if your body can't absorb the nutrients provided. If your gut does not absorb the goodness within the food you feed yourself, all that goodness you fed yourself will just go through the digestive canal and end out the other end. Oh no! Yep, that was my reaction exactly.

With this in mind, we need to look after the gut flora, clean out the garbage and the excess and prepare ourselves to receive. 'You are what you absorb' became a better phrase to live by. I do suggest you 'clean up' a bit, so that you better receive the goodness you put in. Do a gentle detox and then start to incorporate better quality foods into your diet.

Gentle is better than putting your body through a full-on detox that might cause stress within. Clean out what does not serve your body. Listen to how you react to different things and enjoy some detox juices. Cut down on stimulants, like coffee, tea, alcohol, and sugar.

The goal is to find a healthy diet that works for you and your body.

A whole-food diet. I believe we have different needs and preferences based on genetics, culture, intolerances, lifestyle, moral considerations, and personal taste. However, eating a diet that places an emphasis on plant-based options and minimises processed and pre-packaged food is the number one priority. Use your body wisdom and cultivate your ability to work together on your journey.

Plant-based foods contain enzymes that support the digestive process and provide fuel for good bacteria, whilst processed foods tend to be loaded with sugar and chemicals and encourage the overgrowth of bad bacteria in the gut.

Avoid inflammation causing foods – why? Inflammation is one of many causes of illness and disease in your body. Inflammation could have started many years ago – accumulation over time – and there it is! As a result of inflammation, your genes suddenly decide to express themselves as 'something' – an illness or disease, ache, or pain.

Some inflammation causing foods:

- The white stuff - white bread, white potatoes, and SUGAR!
- Processed food - tinned vegetables, savoury snacks like crisps and sausage rolls, cheese
- Vegetable and seed oils - stick to olive oil and coconut oil
- Refined carbohydrates, such as white bread and pastries

Let's Talk About Sugar

There are many types of sugar, and they each have some important differences. Glucose is the type of sugar your body uses for energy.

Brown sugar, versus white sugar: just because brown sugar is the colour of dirt does not make it more natural or healthier than its white counterpart. The colour comes from a common residual sticky syrup, called molasses.

Honey, Golden Syrup: they are all sugar products and equally harmful for us. They all pack kilojoules and calories and not much else in forms of nutrients. FAT does not make you fat; sugar does.

Agave is not a very healthful replacement for table sugar. While it is less harmful and more natural than sugar, people who are closely managing blood glucose should avoid agave. The high fructose content can reduce insulin sensitivity and may worsen liver health. Agave is also a higher-calorie sweetener than table sugar.

Stevia is natural, unlike other sugar substitutes. It's made from a leaf related to popular garden flowers like asters and chrysanthemums. People have been using stevia leaves to sweeten drinks like tea for many years. Stevia is a good sugar substitute, as long as you consume it in moderation. Too much of it may cause gas, nausea, and inflammation in your body.

Supplements to support your body

I am a big believer in supplementation. It is needed on a cellular level to help protect, repair and regenerate. In today's busy world we can't rely on food for our nutrition. It doesn't matter how many organic carrots I buy; it will not match the energy in that carrot I spoke about earlier. That carrot I pulled up from my garden patch as a little girl. This is due to depletion of the nourishment in today's soil. It is impossible for us to consume enough of all the vitamins, minerals, phytochemicals, and everything else your body needs.

I take food supplements and have done so for many years. It gives me the nutrients I need and lifts me to another level of health and wellbeing. Eat good quality food and take good quality supplements to reach your full potential. Choose wisely! I personally have chosen supplements that not only give me the vitamins and minerals I need, but also provides me with Age Defence Mechanism and anti-inflammatory properties.

There are some products that will benefit all of us, and these are products I personally take: a quality fruit and vegetable supplement in combination with a good quality Omega supplement.

Collagen is another product I believe becomes very important as we go through the ageing process. Collagen is basically everywhere in your body and your own collagen production goes down with age.

A Collagen supplement can help make your bones denser, slowing down the ageing process that makes them brittle and help your body produce new bone. Collagen is also in your skin – so a Collagen supplement is nourishing you skin from the inside out. Yes, it has you both looking and feeling younger.

Seasonal food for proper nourishment

Let's go back to the philosophy of macrobiotics. Our goal here is to harmonise ourselves with the movement of the prevailing season. Every season according to Chinese Medicine is connected to certain internal organs and its function. Eating and nourishing yourself in alignment with the seasons will strengthen your internal organs and prepare them for optimal action and performance.

Below are some suggestions for you of foods you might want to incorporate into your diet. Foods that will help energise and recharge your batteries. Work on feeding the energy of your internal organs and organ function to support you to be the best version of You.

The Season of Spring

Liver and Gallbladder correspond to the season of Spring. Spring is the season when the Liver energy is most intense and a wonderful time to pay extra attention to look after it. Spring is also a time of upwards and outgoing energy, time for new life and planning, creativity, and expansion.

Spring cleaning is not only beneficial for our homes and gardens. It is fantastic for your body and mind. I well remember my Shiatsu mentor's words: 'When you want to clean your mind, please, go and clean out your kitchen cupboards.' I have followed this advice and it works wonders. A Spring clean is necessary for your body and especially the liver. This is a great time to let go of any extra stimulants, as the spring energy will give you that boost naturally. Focus on a cleansing diet rich in vegetables and fresh fruit.

Examples of recommended foods for the spring, your Liver and Gallbladder energy include

– onions, leeks, leaf mustard,
– Chinese yam, dates,
– mushrooms,
– spinach and bamboo shoots.
– fresh green and leafy vegetables should also be included in meals.
– sprouts from seeds are also valuable.
– bananas, pears, water chestnuts, celery, and cucumber

Summertime

When living in accordance with Nature's Rhythms, this is the time of the year when you are in full flow. Expansive, outwards going, fully expressed, and living full out, unapologetically! Joy is in the air, it is warm outside, the sun is out shining on you. Everything in nature grows quickly and vitality is high. The energy is buzzing. And so are you, your body and mind.

Summer nourishes our Heart and Small Intestine energy. The heart circulates oxygen-rich blood and assures proper assimilation in the small intestine. When the heart is balanced, the mind tends to calm down. We sleep profoundly, wake up in the early morning hours, nicely rested with the energy we need.

This is the time of the year when it is extra important to drink plenty of water to cool and hydrate yourself. Indulge in delicious salads filled with raw vegetables and enjoy some seafood in the mix. Choose pungent flavours and reduce the bitter taste. Choose frequently from the below list:

- Cucumber, bok choy, broccoli, asparagus
- Tomatoes, lemon, and sprouts
- Watermelon, strawberries, peach, and orange
- Spinach, Summer squash, and bean sprouts
- Fish

Autumn is here…

In Autumn things need to turn inwards a bit, in preparation for the winter. The long summer days become shorter, and we start to dress in warmer clothes. The dryer weather can cause a sore throat, a dry nose, chest infections, rough skin, hair loss, and dry stools. We need to eat to promote the production of body fluids and their lubricating effects throughout the body.

Autumn time is harvesting time. Longer cooking times and heartier food will be beneficial foods to support your immune system and set yourself up for the winter season. Enjoy making plenty of soups and stews which are warming and easier to digest for your body.

- nuts or seeds, like walnuts and almonds
- pumpkin, sweet potato
- onion and leeks
- radish, broccoli and asparagus
- cardamom, chili, and cinnamon
- pears, banana, and apricots
- cucumber, celery, and sauerkraut
- eggs and olives
- pickles, lemons, vinegar
- lemon and limes
- apples, grapes, and plums

Winter - Time to Slow Down and Draw Inwards

In winter, living things slow down to save energy. Some animals in cooler areas, like my home country, Sweden, decide to hibernate. It is also the season where humans conserve energy and build strength as a prelude to spring.

This is a great time of the year to eat warmer food, soups, and more cooked food to warm our body and spirit. Consume appropriate fats and high protein foods. This is Kidney time of the year – most black foods nourish the Kidney energy. Water is necessary for your Kidneys to thrive, so keep hydrating well, please.

- lettuce, watercress, endives
- asparagus, celery
- miso, soya sauce, seaweed, kale
- warm hearty soups
- small dark beans, kidney beans!
- include ginger in your food
- roasted nuts and dried foods
- steamed winter greens
- quinoa
- bone broth

One bite at a time!

I love food! I love eating food that has been prepared and cooked with love and intention. It tastes so much better, and I can feel the energy from the food really nourishing me and my body. Please take time when you prepare your food. Bring some love and joy into the process and focus on the task at hand.

Have fun trying out different dishes and recipes. Include all the different colours into it. Red for summer, black for winter, green for spring, and white for the autumn time. Present it nicely and create space and time around eating it. Chew well and allow yourself time to really taste it. Rushing a meal is not going to give you the energy you want. Slow down, sit down, and enJOY!

Moving with JOY

"If it doesn't challenge you, it doesn't change you."

Fred Derito

Exercise with focus and intent and cultivate the love of moving your body – is that possible, you might ask? Sure, it is, and I do encourage you to move more. The beauty of this challenge is that you get to choose what movement feels right for you. With challenge comes growth, and I invite you to take time to create new practices in your day aligned with your intentions and goals, that help you to become the best version of you. Commit to not only move your body more, but to prioritise You, and I promise, your body will thank you for it.

Movement is Medicine

I'm a bit of an exercise devotee. Yep, I love being active and moving my body. It is a great outlet for me. It helps me clear my mind, sort my thoughts, and helps me deal better with any daily little stressors' life has on offer. The truth is, I don't feel well if I don't move.

Exercise has so many health benefits, so when working on upping your game and being the best, most vibrant version of You, it becomes a necessary ingredient.

Exercise releases endorphins in the brain. Endorphins are peptide hormones with similar effects as morphine. In other words, a natural and safe 'high.' So, exercise produces happy feelings within, which helps you to stay on track of achieving your intentions and goals around your health and wellbeing.

Good mobility is also the key to maintaining healthy joints and a pain-free body. With age, you gradually lose range of motion, strength, and flexibility when you don't stay on top of it. Too often we take for granted our ability to easily move around and function in daily life. Movement helps create more space and joint freedom, all while strengthening weak and underused muscles, and eliminating pain.

'Motion is lotion' and keeping your body moving is the greatest way to prevent age-related physical issues. My Pilates studio has a saying on the wall as we enter, saying 'Movement is Medicine,' and I agree. In so many ways this is true. Becoming healthy is the best decision I ever made.

'But I don't like exercising…' you might say. The trick is to find a type of movement/exercise that you enjoy and keep doing it. Movement that have you looking forward to your training session and that gives your body what it needs at the same time. When choosing, remember to choose an exercise according to your age – I can't do the same type of exercise today and push myself as I did when I was younger. My body will scream loudly if I do. Balance and moderation are the key.

In Sweden there is a word: lagom. 'Lagom' best translates as 'just right'— not too much and not too little and just the right amount. Different to balance and closely related. While there is something admirable about training hard to improve fitness levels, there is a fine line between that and pushing yourself to extremes.

I have been there, and it doesn't work long term. Too much of anything causes stress within and your body will complain. You will burn out. The trick is to look for the 'lagom' amount. Fitness training and exercise should be enjoyable, not causing stress; but at the same time, you want results, a bit of challenge to create the change you are looking for.

My parents put me into acrobatics as a five-year-old girl. Acrobatics became gymnastics a couple of years later, and I believe they did this for me to have an outlet for my excess energy. I spent many hours in the gymnasium during my school years and have wonderful memories of the comradeship in our Gymnastic Team.

The encouragement and all the uplifting comments during the tough times and the celebration and enjoyment when successes were there. Exercise fills so many more areas of fulfilment in our life on top of keeping fit and strong.

I trained to become a physical education teacher back in Sweden. This gave me the opportunity to try many ways of movement and exercise. Not all the time out of choice, I should add. It was all part of the training.

For example, if you want to be a P.E. teacher in Sweden, you need to know how to do downhill skiing in case you end up as a teacher up in the northern part of the country. Well, I did not mind that one at all. I loved it. It was great fun and I excelled at it. Many trips down to the Alps followed and downhill skiing has been a big part of my life, but I must say ice hockey was not one of my favourite lessons.

The truth is, we as humans were not meant to sit down all day long, but unfortunately that is what many of us are doing due to the sedentary lifestyles we have. Our body was meant to move and be active. As a young girl, I walked, used my push bike, and in the winter, I skied to school. That is unusual today – instead we drive our kids to school or drop them at the bus stop. In today's world we need to seek time and space in our day to move our body.

Some of us need it more than others, all depending on what your life looks like, what kind of work you do. A young mother with small children doing housework and shopping needs different type of exercise than a woman sitting on an office chair all day long. A gardener or carpenter, physically using his/her body all day long, is not in the need of the same type of exercise as the accountant or bank manager. But we all need to MOVE to enhance our vitality and stay healthy.

- Move to keep all the systems within function the way they should.
- Move to stay fit and strong enough to enjoy life.
- Move to keep flexible in body and mind.
- Move to help shift the food we take on.
- Move to help our mind to quiet down, and
- Move to lift our moods.

Find Your Own Love of Moving

Walking and swimming are great ways of getting yourself up and moving. A very safe way to exercise, and both will increase your heartbeat and work some of your muscles. To do it together with others will add a social component to it and probably hold you accountable in a better way. As well as keeping you motivated, being in a group puts a smile on your face and adds value to your life with the social connection. A sense of belonging and human connection are vital parts of your health and longevity.

Look at using everyday opportunities to move. Could you combine your need for movement with something else? Take time to walk around during your lunch break. Park the car a bit away from your work and walk the last bit. Take the stairs instead of the elevator. Semi-strenuous, everyday tasks performed regularly can help keep you fit and healthy. If you like me, like to run, that can do wonders for your mental clarity and your general mood, but only if you don't overdo it.

Dancing is something I love and another wonderful way to exercise. I used to do lots of this when I lived in New York. I went to different kind of dance studios, placed myself in the back of the class working myself through the routines, trying not to tangle myself up too much. Music helped and I had FUN! Was I brilliant at it? No way, but it did not matter.

What mattered was I moved and enjoyed myself. I focused, sweated, laughed, and felt fabulous afterwards. There are so many various forms of dancing to try: belly dancing, ballroom dancing, salsa, African dancing, pole dancing. The list is long, and it is just about being a little bit daring and trying. Maybe this is the type of exercise you will start to love.

Harmonise Body and Mind

I now practice Yoga regularly myself and love the positive benefits it gives me and my body. Yoga practice stills my mind and has me focus within. It stretches and moves my body, muscles, and energy channels allowing the energy to flow more freely. Life energy flows through us like a swift stream when there is nothing to obstruct it. In Yoga we use physical movements, called asanas, together with breath awareness, pranayama in our practice session. Most classes bring in meditation to help with focus in the Yoga practice and some schools include internalisation and ethical observances to help reach that state of union or harmony called 'samadhi.' A beautiful, still place to experience.

The traditional translation of yoga is 'union.' Yoga promotes union of body, mind, and spirit, which leads to a greater sense of harmony and peace, not only within us, but also in our interactions with others and the world around us. Although 'Samadhi' is a goal, we first experience improved health, greater ease in our body, and we start to feel more relaxed, more centered, and naturally calmer within.

Everyone who practices Yoga will benefit in one way or the other, and the beauty is that Yoga practice can easily be adapted to any age, body shape, and fitness level. I use Yoga as a way of feeling connected – connected to my body, mind, and spirit and in a greater sense of interconnectedness of all things.

Different Types of Yoga:

There are many different types of yoga available, whether you want a more physically demanding class or an easy, relaxing, meditative class. With each style being a bit different from the others, you'll find variations depending on the teacher. I recommend giving a few styles and teachers a try before deciding which style to go for.

- *Hatha Yoga* - the Sanskrit term 'hatha' refers to any yoga that teaches physical postures. Hatha Yoga is a practice of the body, a physical practice where you will hold your posture for a few breaths, before moving to the next. Hatha Yoga is considered a gentler form of Yoga and a great start if you are a beginner.
- *Vinyasa Yoga* - a more dynamic Yoga practice that links movement and breath together in a dance-like way. Some teachers will add music to the practice. You will not linger too long in each posture, allowing your heart rate to rise.
- *Ashtanga Yoga* - a bit more challenging practice, where you will flow and breathe through each pose to build internal heat. In Ashtanga Yoga we perform the same poses in the exact same order in each class. This is one of my favourite types of Yoga – it does challenge me and has me really focus on my breath throughout the practice.
- *Iyengar Yoga* - we bring great importance to our body's alignment in each pose. Different helpful props, from yoga blocks and blankets to straps or a ropes wall, will become your

new best friend, helping you to work within a range of motion that is safe and effective for you.

- *Bikram Yoga* - Here you practice a set sequence of postures in a heated, humid environment. The heat can be challenging and strenuous, so start easy. Important to be hydrated and as a beginner, take it easy to start with.
- *Yin Yoga* - This is a more meditative practice and designed to target your deeper connective tissues and fascia, restoring length and elasticity. In Yin yoga the different poses are held for several minutes at a time, supporting you to calm and balance your body and mind. Some will say, this is the practice where you will find your Zen.
- *Restorative Yoga* - Great for anyone who has a hard time relaxing and slowing down! The slow-moving practice and longer holds allow you and your body a chance tap into your parasympathetic nervous system and experience a deeper relaxation. You might also use various props for support and getting into poses.
- *Kundalini Yoga* - Good for people looking for a most spiritual Yoga practice. You will perform repetitive physical exercises, called 'kriyas,' combined with intense breathwork. Chanting, singing, and meditation is also

part of the Kundalini practice. The aim is to help you break through any internal barriers, to release any untapped energy residing within, allowing you a greater level of self-awareness.

Plenty of choices, so no excuses! Check what is available in your area, try a few different classes and teachers and see what and which one resonates with you. Stick with it for a few weeks and dedicate to your practice. You will improve by the class and start to feel the various benefits; and if it does not resonate any longer, try another class. Incorporating a variety of types of yoga into your regular practice can help keep you balanced.

Elongate Your Muscles and Restore

The last couple of years I have enjoyed bringing in Pilates into my movement routine. I love working out on the reformer machines. Great for keeping fit and strong throughout my ageing process as we work with resistance all the time on the reformers. Pilates Reformer training is a brilliant way of strengthening your core muscles.

> *"A strong core will improve your technique, strength, and stamina, and compliment everything you do."*
>
> **Susan Trainor**

Below are five great benefits with practising Reformer Pilates:

1. It gives you a balanced, full body workout. The subtly of the springs on a Reformer strengthens the whole body to target the large muscle movers and activate the smaller stabilisers at the same time.

2. Low impact - high intensity. The springs are specifically designed to enable you to work in the horizontal plane rather than weight-bearing. This reduces the load through your body. The low impact allows for repetitive movements to occur which in turn tones and strengthens any injured areas to speed recovery.

3. Improved posture and core strength. Many of the exercises performed on a Reformer machine target the core whilst working the peripheral postural muscles at the same time.

4. Tones muscles and builds strength. Reformer Pilates have you move through full range while working on strengthening muscles. It uses the machine's springs and levers to create resistance and allow for equal focus on the concentric and eccentric contractions to create long, lean, toned muscles.

5. Improves your mental health and wellbeing. How is this possible, you may ask? From focusing of your breath to find mindfulness

in movement to stress management and relaxation. Reformer Pilates, like other physical exercise, can reduce stress hormones like cortisol. It can increase endorphins, your body's feel-good chemicals, giving you a natural mood boost.

To complete this section, here is another benefit of exercise for you – it can improve brain function and protect memory and thinking skills. To begin with, it increases your heart rate, which promotes the flow of blood and oxygen to your brain. It can also stimulate the production of hormones that enhance the growth of brain cells.

Plus, exercise enhances your ability to prevent chronic disease that can translate into benefits for your brain, since its function can be affected by these conditions.

Don't have a daily movement routine yet? We look at how to create this in Part 6. We will bring it in as one of your Healthy Habits in combination with all the above. With all the tools in your tool kit, let's look at how you can implement this into your daily life, create a ritual that works for you and gets you to the standard you want to achieve. Not all in one go but one Healthy Habit at a time to avoid failure and disappointment. Keep in mind….

The difference between the body you have and the body you want, are simply the choices you make.

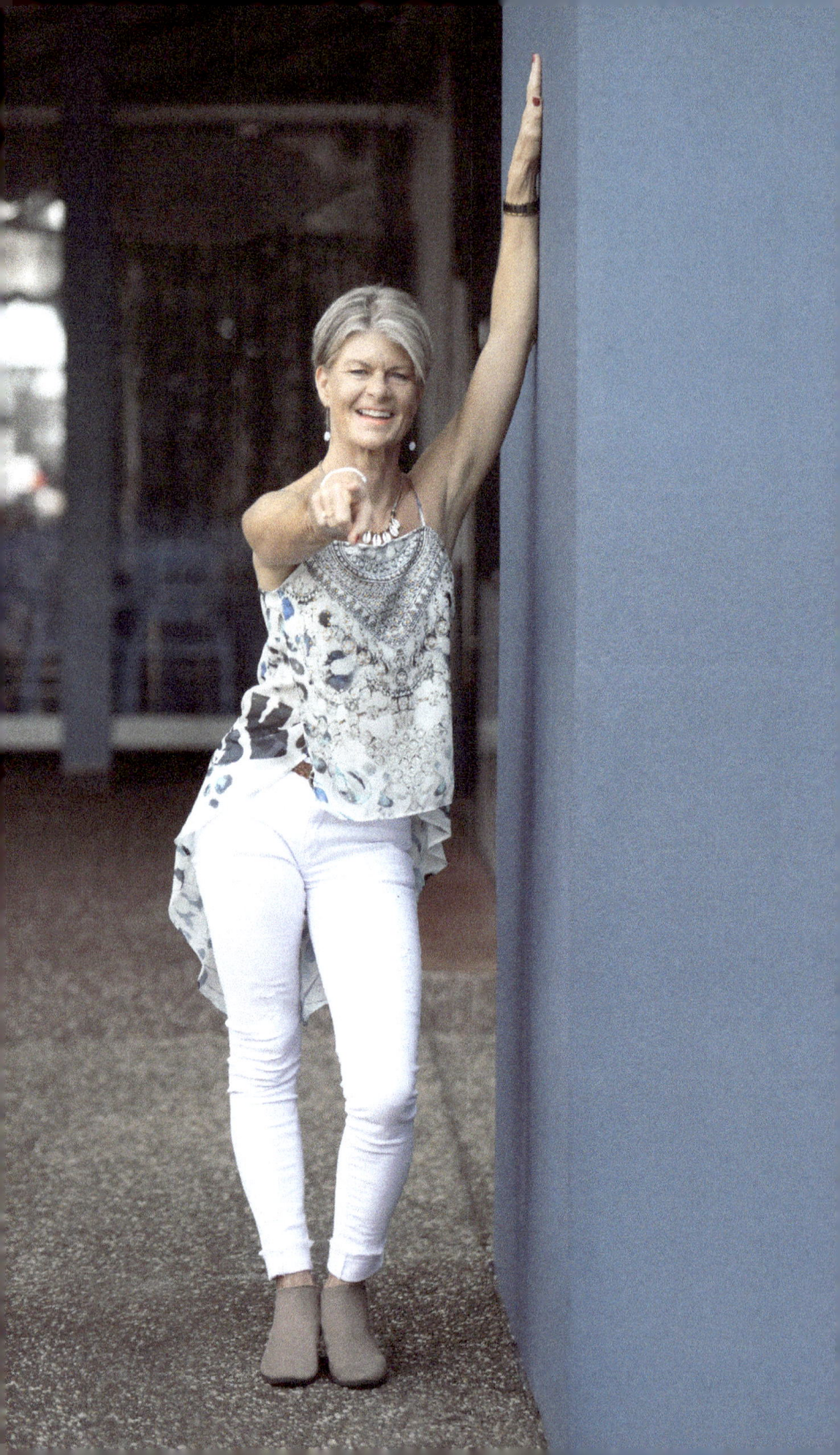

A Positive Attitude

'Attitude is a little thing that makes a big difference.'

Winston Churchill

What does attitude have to do with your health and wellbeing? Everything. Like Mr. Churchill says – it's the little things that make a huge difference.

According to the dictionary, the term 'attitude' refers to an individual's mental state, which is based on his/her beliefs or value system, emotions, and the tendency to act in a certain way. Your attitude reflects in how you think, feel, and behave in any given situation.

Attitude can be defined as your response to people and places, to things or events in your life. It can be referred to as your viewpoint and your mindset, your beliefs, etc. Your attitude towards people, places, things, or situations determines the choices that you make in life. Attitude is composed of three components.

- cognitive component,
- affective/emotional component, and
- behavioural component.

The cognitive component is basically based on information or knowledge you have. The affective component is based on your feelings. The behavioural component reflects how the attitude affects the way you act or behave. I believe that with a positive attitude, life is much easier, and you will have more fun moments in life. Be endlessly curious, take risks, and cultivate a youthful and passionate mind.

"Making each moment count positively is all that life demands from you."

Edmond Mbiaka

Choose Your Thoughts Carefully

"You can't afford the luxury of a negative thought."

John Roger & Peter McWilliams

This is the heading of one of the very first self-development books I picked up when I lived in London. It is written by John-Roger and Peter McWilliams and has the subheading:

'A Book for People with Any Life-Threatening Illness - Including Life'

In the introduction of this very interesting book, it is stated that the book isn't just for people with life threatening illnesses, but a book for 'anyone afflicted with one of the primary diseases of our time: negative thinking.'

According to the authors, negative thinking is always 'expensive' - dragging us down mentally, emotionally, and physically. Hence, they refer to any indulgence in it as a luxury. If, however, they say, you have symptoms of a life-threatening illness - 'negative thinking is a luxury you can't afford.'

In every given moment we have a choice. I choose to start every day with a positive mind. Every day is a new fresh start in my world. On the banner I created for my 'Daring & Disruptive' Female Entrepreneurs Tribe it says, 'Today I choose Happiness.'

An easy choice for me and totally in alignment with my passion in life – to support people to be happy and healthy. Happiness is something you can choose. Happiness is a sense of well-being, joy, or contentment. Not given to you by someone or something else but found within you; a choice – your choice. I choose happiness daily.

Your attitude determines how you choose to response to situations in life. Living in London, me and my husband ran a very successful Shiatsu training organisation called the British School of Shiatsu-Do. We had over 250 students and 25 teachers to look after. Yes, office staff on top of that.

Every three months it was time to pay the government tax, VAT. Ray, my husband, oversaw this and every time it came around to pay, he would complain about the huge amount to pay out. My response: the more we get asked to pay, just means we have done well and influenced more people with the benefit of Shiatsu. We both got the same message but had two different responses.

Choose Your Thoughts Carefully

I like the below poem, called **A New Day:**

*This is the beginning of a new day.
I have been given this day to use as I will.
I can waste it or use it for good.
But what I do today is important,
Because I am exchanging a day of my life for it.
When tomorrow comes, this day will be gone forever,
Leaving in its place something I have traded for it.
I want it to be gain and not loss,
Good and not evil; success and not failure.
In order that I shall not regret the price that
I have paid for it.*

Unknown

The Key to Positive Input

Every experience influences our life one way or the other. We metabolise everything we encounter - physically and emotionally. So, every experience in life becomes a part not only of our minds, but also of our bodies.

Negative experiences are metabolised differently than positive experiences. If you overload the system with negative input, it goes out of balance. The inner harmony is disturbed.

If you substitute positive inputs instead, these also get metabolised into your overall wellbeing, energy level, and health. The best inputs are those experiences that have you feeling lighter both physically and emotionally. From the freshest organic foods, to laughter, to the beauty of nature. Positive input strengthens you on every level, making it much easier to rid your system of toxins.

"Day by day, what you choose, what you think and what you do is who you become."

Heraclitus

Journal Writing

"Those who don't believe in magic will never find it."

Roald Dahl

I started to write my first Gratitude Journal after meeting Dr. Carol McCall at a women's course in the US. The course was called 'The Possibility of Women.' It was a course I went away from with lots of wonderful tools and new skills to implement in my life. One of those was to write acknowledgements to myself daily and to start Journal Writing.

The course had a huge, positive impact on me, and since then I write in my Gratitude Journal every day. If you never done this before, I highly recommend you get started. Gratitude is simple, yet so profound. Whilst it is not a Magic Pill, there is certainly some magic at work here. Some people will say it is the simplest, most effective thing you can do every day to be happier. And it has been proven that shifting your focus to the positive can dramatically improve your happiness. The key is consistency.

I suggest you go out and buy yourself that special little notebook to write in. Then place it next to your bed, on your bedside table, together with a pen.

Why? It will remind you of writing in it first thing in the morning and last thing at night. Once you start, you can't stop. Once the habit is created, you will 'need' to do it before starting you day and before falling asleep.

Gratitude derives from the Latin word gratia meaning grace, graciousness, or gratefulness. It is really the feeling that embodies the words 'Thank You.' There are so many great benefits with writing a Gratitude Journal. Harvard Health contends that "gratitude helps people feel more positive emotions, relish good experiences, improve their health, deal with adversity, and build strong relationships."

Yep, Magic at work! It strengthens your immune system and connectedness to others, increases endorphin, serotonin and dopamine levels and your ability to cope with pain and stress. Improved sleep. The list is long, so let's get started.

You can choose what to focus on every day of your life. So, take your Gratitude Journal, choose a quiet place to sit and spend five minutes in the beginning of your day to decide what you want to focus on that day. Start by writing down three things you are grateful for today. This can be things you already have experienced in your life, or things you not yet have in your life.

Challenge yourself to write down different things every day. Very soon you will realise that there is plenty to be grateful for in your life. The sun shining from a clear blue sky. Maybe the rain falling, nourishing

Journal Writing

mother nature. Waking up in a wonderful, warm bed after a deep night's sleep. Or the relationship you are looking for and yet do not have – I am grateful to be in a nourishing, loving relationship with the partner of my dreams.

You can also program your mind by writing down a few sentences on 'today what would make a great day?' Have a think and then write down three things that would create a better day for you. Important here is that you are in control over the things you write down. When I was in the process of writing this book, I wrote down 'create time for me to write my book.' Another example: making time to go for a walk on the beach; increased action in my business; a successful business appointment…

Finish up with an affirmation – a 'I am statement'…I am happy in my skin, I am confident, I am excited…. A statement of what you want in life. I am committed, I am hopeful and trusting the Journey. Something that resonates with you and sets you up with a nice focus for the day. By doing this you prime your brain to start building this belief in your mind. And with consistency, you will begin to create the change from within. Be consistent and persistent and trust the process.

At the very end of the day, please go back to your Journal. Evening time is the time for reflection. Reflect on your day and draw out the three amazing things that happened. Unexpected and expected positive happenings in your day. It can be that wonderful cup of coffee you had. Or the business deal that finally went through. Seeing your daughter/son performing well at sports day in school. Having time to be you. Whatever it is, write down the highlights of your day in your Journal.

You are priming your brain by going to sleep with positive things in your mind. This will occupy your unconscious mind during you sleep and yes, Gratitude as mentioned before will help improve your sleep. As part of this reflection time, you can also add something you learned during the day. What 'aha' moment/s did you have during your day? Reflect on every aspect of your day and ask yourself the question: what went fabulously well, and where can I make some improvements?

I used to do this after my teaching days as a P.E. teacher back in Sweden. I wanted to excel and be the best possible teacher and mentor for my students and the reflection times became a big part of getting me there. In our Shiatsu school we asked our students for feedback on their classes content and the teacher. Great to hear their reflection and vitally important to do your own reflection before reading their feedback.

Please act and make magic happen. Commit to five consecutive days to start with and stick with it. In time, it will grow into a nice, rewarding habit.

> *"Never go to sleep without a request to your subconscious."*
>
> **Thomas Edison**

Mindfulness Meditation

> *"The road to health for everyone is through moderation, harmony, and a sound mind in a sound body."*
>
> **Jostein Gaarder**

I don't know how many times I have heard and read that meditation is good for you. I kept asking the question 'in what terms' is it beneficial for me and my body and are there good scientific studies showing specific benefits that I care about? And the answer is yes, there are plenty of them and the message is the same: 15 - 20 minutes of daily meditation and inner stillness will help you find your true nature and discover your path to health and happiness. It is in stillness you will discover your soul's purpose and create a life in which all things are within reach.

Total Balance Is Natural Balance

If we understand that some sort of balance in our life is desirable, it will elude us if we approach balance with different parts of our life separately. Because all the pieces are interconnected, it's better to look at the whole mind-body system. If you're aiming for balance, you cannot achieve this by struggle, or fighting with yourself. I did and it did not work. I avoided meditation and had all different kind of excuse for not sitting down and being still. Told myself my running was my meditation practice.

Yes, running has me focused and quiets my mind to a certain extent, but my energy is needed for the movement my body is using. This was not allowing the focus on inner peace and finding out about my true self. Meditation will help take me there. In meditation you find your true self, and as you continue the practice, you identify with it more and more. And the beautiful thing, with time, is that you will discover that you were whole all along.

In meditation, we reach the quiet, centred place within that does not hold on to toxic habits. This is when old behaviour and letting go of emotional baggage happens naturally.

There are many ways to meditate, and you might already be practising some form yourself. There is no form that is better than the other. Any kind of authentic meditation will include the positive benefits listed below. Evidence do show that the practice will be more beneficial for you if you find a technique that you really like, and you will if that is what you want. You will know when you have found it, as you will enjoy and even look forward to your daily practice.

Benefits of Meditation:

- Meditation might help you live longer
- Meditation helps manage your heart rate and respiratory rate
- Meditation reduces the sense of loneliness, heart disease, and depression
- Meditation helps treat menopausal problems and premenstrual syndrome
- Meditation is effective in relieving breathing problems like asthma and other inflammatory bowel disorders
- Meditation help reduce blood pressure
- Meditation affects genes that control stress and immunity. It prepares you to deal with stressful events in a better way
- Meditation increases awareness of your unconscious mind
- Meditation improves your memory
- Meditation improves your mood and emotional wellbeing
- Meditation helps your focus, attention and ability to concentrate at the task at hand
- Meditation reduces emotional eating
- Meditation increase feelings of compassion and reduces worry
- Meditation improves positive relationship and feelings of empathy

The list is long and there is so much more to add. Meditation will keep you healthy and happier on all levels, but it takes daily practice and your commitment to get there. The result you are aiming for with your meditation practice is mindfulness. Mindfulness throughout your day, in any given moment. Mindfulness is about being present and living each moment in your life with full attention.

Time to find your space for stillness, so you can get on and sense the above benefits bit by bit. I'm not telling you this will be an easy journey, but maybe it will be. I struggled to start with but when I finally found my space to sit and be quiet, I thoroughly enjoyed it. The space is a beautiful one to visit. An inner space where you allow yourself to just be, wonder within, and become aware of your true self.

Where to find the time, you might ask yourself. I think most of us can relate to not having enough time in life and the amazing thing is, we find we have more time when we meditate because we become more productive. If 20 minutes feels too much to start with, do 10, or even 5 minutes per day. The important thing is you get on and just do it. Even one or two minutes of meditation each day could make a world of difference in your emotional state and mindset.

Many will say that the morning hours is the best time to meditate, as soon as you get out of bed and have taken care of your bodily function. It will set you up for the day ahead and bring your peaceful state of mind into the rest of your day. Maybe you are already waking up early and can fit your meditation time in, before starting your daily activities. Maybe you need to set your alarm to wake up 15 minutes earlier in the morning. Some choose to do their practice at the end of the day. Once again, the important thing is to decide, pick a time, same time every day, and just get started.

To start with, my space for stillness was on the beach, outside where I could hear the waves and the sound of the wind. To meditate and seek inner stillness in nature works for me and I fit my stillness time into what I call my 'Miracle Morning.'

I have also created a small space in my house where I can sit and do my practice. The space in my house has a few items around that help me with my focus. Small things I enjoy having close by - my meditation pillow to sit on, a small Buddha figure, a nice candle, and a few crystals supporting the energy I want to create for myself. All little things that support me in calming down, tuning in and feeling safe in my space.

Below is a short and easy breathing practice that will help you settle and prepare you for meditation practice. The focus you give to your breath will help you find your inner stillness and peace. Follow with sitting still, breathing normally in and out through your nose, and enJOY!

- Begin by sitting in a comfortable cross-legged position on your meditation pillow – lotus if you can – or sit on a chair with your feet firmly on the ground. Lift up from the top of your head and feel your spine nice and straight, allowing energy to flow freely up and down your back. Relax your shoulders and gently tuck your chin in, without straining your neck.

- Start by taking a few deep breaths in through your nose and out through your mouth. Then begin your 'Alternate Nostril Breathing.' This is a wonderful practice that will quickly and effectively calm your nervous system and reduce stress in your body.

- With one hand, use your thumb, ring, and little finger to alternatively close each of your nostrils. The other two fingers can be curled into the palm of your hand or resting on your forehead. Start by exhaling everything out through both nostrils. Then inhale just through your right nostril and closing the other nostril with your fingers or thumb. Then exhale through your left nostril closing the right one.

- Then inhale through the left and breathe out through the right. Switch every time when you are at the top of your inhalation, please. Practice this slowly for a few minutes, then relax your arms in your lap and breathe normally again. Yes, you will most likely find your breathing has calmed down and become deeper already, enhancing your meditation practice further.

"Take a deep breath. Inhale peace. Exhale Happiness."

A D Posey

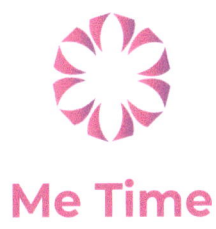

Me Time

"Alone time is when I distance myself from the voices of the world so, I can hear my own."

Oprah

Is it important for your mind, body, and soul to take time out of your busy schedule?

If so, why?

Psychologists have demonstrated that taking some alone time helps to reboot our brains. Time alone improves our concentration and productivity in the long term and helps us to relax and unwind. So, the answer to the question above is a big YES! ME time is important. It's not selfish to take 'me time.' It is the opposite as it better equips us for future social interaction. In my opinion it is a necessity.

Most of us have been on a plane at some stage in our life. And we have all heard the flight attendant taking us through the guidelines if there is an accident. What do they say about the mask dropping down from the ceiling? Put it on your own face first, then help other people. If you do not look after you, you will run out of steam and not be able to be there for your nearest and dearest. Me-sponsible! I love this 'new' word in my vocabulary.

'ME-sponsible'

- the act of being responsible to ME for the benefit of my health, happiness, and wellbeing -

The most common excuse for not creating ME time among the people I meet is lack of time. Time is the most equal thing in this world. We all have the same amount of it – 24 hours a day, every hour 60 minutes, and every minute 60 seconds long. 'I don't have time' is just that – an excuse. It is not about time; it is about priorities. If ME-time is a priority, you will create the time for it in your day. In my opinion, alone time should be high on your priority list.

I think we need to schedule alone time in as though it's as important as any other appointments or meetings in your day. Even just closing your eyes for five minutes and concentrating on taking deep breaths can be all it takes to reap the benefits. I work with many mothers who create ME-time in the end of their busy day.

Closing the bathroom door, draw a bath, look after their body, light a candle, be still, and empty their mind for a few minutes. Starting small and work it from there. Once they start doing it and feeling the benefits, they keep going. It 'pays back' plentiful.

My best time for ME-time is first thing in the morning. I don't have children around anymore and this is my choice and what works for me. You will find your time and work it from there. The important thing is to do it. Five minutes a day to start with and expand from there. Maybe those five minutes is after you dropped your kids to school – still sitting in the car. Close your eyes and take five to ten minutes for you to restore. The rest of the day will move in a better flow when you do.

ME-time is the space you need to reconnect with your inner essence. This is when you give yourself the opportunity to reconnect to your inner vitality, the unlimited energy, creativity, and health that naturally resides in you. When you connect to that inner essence, you have so much more to give to others. So, it is not only an investment in you, but ultimately in the people you love, and I can't see any selfishness in that.

Inner Essence, Purpose, and Bliss

Creating an inspiring purpose for you and your life is the fuel you need to move you from where you are to where you want to go. Everyone has a unique purpose in life. You have a powerful purpose in life. To realise your purpose is the key to fulfil your creative potential. When there is alignment between your purpose, your goals and intentions, and your actions – that's when you live and fulfil your full potential.

My Body and Me

"True happiness comes through reaching for your full potential."

When you live on purpose, nothing or no one can really stop you. You are clear about where you are going and what actions you need to take. Your purpose is your 'Why?' – it is your spark. No challenge, difficulty, or obstacle can get in your way. You feel excited by what's possible, and life is in flow. People will start to notice the change in your energy, and you slowly start to transform your life, and by doing so, the life of those around you.

When you feel positive about yourself and know that you are actively maintaining a healthy lifestyle, it will reflect in your appearance. Knowing that you are doing the best for yourself and enjoying the process will bring a healthy glow to your skin, both physically and metaphorically. 'Feel good – look good!' And yes, you will soon become aware of the benefits of having greater vitality simply from the way people look at you: that spark of life twinkling in your eyes will express self-confidence and security.

This self-confidence will help in both your personal life and career, enabling you to release your potential and live life to the fullest. As you fulfil your purpose and unlock more of your body and mind's potential, you will naturally feel happier, content, and even blissful.

Me Time

'Follow your bliss' – what does that expression really mean? Following your bliss means trusting that everything will work out, even if things aren't completely perfect. Success will come at some point, but not necessarily right away or the way you thought it would. Universe provides in the most mysterious ways sometimes. The more you give, the more you receive.

When you follow your bliss, you put yourself on a path that has been there all the time, just waiting for you. Wherever you are, if you are following your bliss, you are enjoying that refreshment, that life within you, all the time.

"With each step...
we arrive at our destination.
Because right there, right now,
is where we're supposed to be."

Source Unknown

Self-love - the Gift that Keeps on Giving

"To Love Oneself is the beginning of a lifelong romance."

Oscar Wilde

- Do you say yes when you really mean no?
- Do you break promises to yourself or neglect your self-care?
- Do you put yourself first?

It is common, especially among women, to put other people's needs in front of our own. And if this, is you, it is time to give yourself the most important gift ever: self-love.

The truth is, before you can receive love and respect from others, you need to love and respect yourself. And the good news is when you love yourself fully, you feed your soul and become the highest version of you. It feels natural to take good care of your body, mind, and spirit. You have the energy to give, and in turn, giving energises you. Everyone benefits. As cliché as it sounds, self-love is the gift that keeps on giving.

My Body and Me

Love yourself for who you are. Comparing yourself with others doesn't serve. Loving yourself provides you with self-confidence, self-worth, and in general you will feel more positive. A healthy sense of self-love and self-care provide you with the strength to be the light for others.

If you are at a place in life where you must hide parts of yourself to get along, please start to make the necessary changes so that you can be your true, authentic self everywhere you go.

You are far more powerful than you ever dreamed. As you discover and learn how to use your power, please use it for your own upliftment and the upliftment of others.

You are a marvelous, wonderful, worthwhile person – just because you are! That's my viewpoint, and I invite you to join me for a while at that viewing point.

> *"Life is a journey, and if you fall in love with the journey, you will be in love forever."*
>
> **Peter Hagerty**

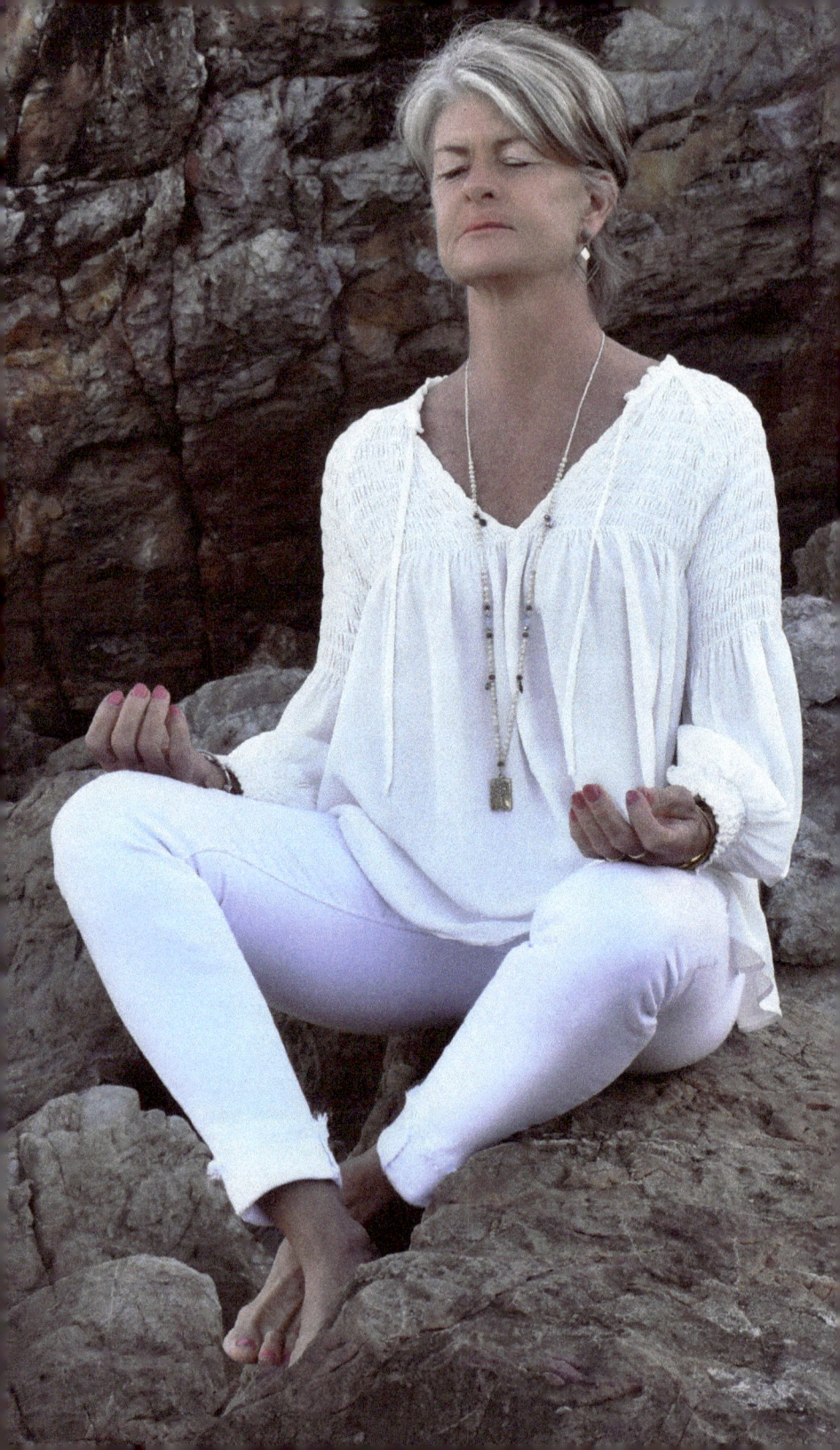

Listening

"One of the most sincere forms of respect is actually listening to what another has to say."

Bryant H. McGill

Listening is one of the most empowering tools in communication, but it has been given the least credit. Listening is the nucleus of real communication. When we listen, we also become powerful speakers. Listening can be proactive, and as an empowered listener, you can become an empowered speaker and make your voice heard. It is time to shift what we call your 'Automatic Reactive Listening' to 'Empowered Listening.'

Attentive listening is a beautiful and powerful skill, the product of a paradigm shift that allows you to enter a partnership with the speaker. When you listen unconditionally, without judgment and criticism, you will get to hear a person's truth. Trust and intimacy begin to happen; the speaker begins to open and speak from their depth.

The Healing Power of Listening

"Listen, there is a world out there waiting to be heard."

Carol McCall

I spent a few years studying with Dr. Carol McCall, a beautiful woman, and a coach in Listening and Communication. Dr. Carol based her work on scientific research showing that when we are truly being heard, our body releases endorphins – neurotransmitters creating 'happy' feelings in your body.

When you take the time to truly listen to the person you have a conversation with, you are providing a healing space for that person. Truly listening means listening from your heart, not just your ears. Yes, we do have two ears and one mouth, and it is wonderful when we use them accordingly.

This type of listening requires your full attention. It requires you to be totally present in the moment, without anything else distracting you from your listening. What happens most of the time though, is that you are busily thinking about something else – your next activity, what's happening at home, the shopping you are supposed to do. Your mind shifts to other things, and you don't 'hear' what is being said. We all have our 'Automatic Listening' style and I'm sure you can relate to some of the ones listed below:

When someone speaks, this might be what's going on in your head…

- I have heard it before…
- Been there, done that…
- When is she coming to the point…. hurry up!
- Rather than listening, you are thinking of what you are going to say next…
- Future thinking…. not here…

When you truly listen, the above does not happen. Instead, you allow the person you are talking to, to feel that they are being heard. They relax, start to open, to talk and share from within. They unravel things for themselves, come to realisations, solutions. You are providing a space for that person to discover on a deeper level. It's a Journey of Discovery!

The same is true when you listen to your heart and your own heart's desire. You start to realise new ways of doing things, alternative solutions, and you discover deeper truths about you. Unfortunately, many of us do not listen to that inner voice, our heart and intuition. Instead, we listen to our intellectual mind, that voice telling you that you cannot do this or that. Who are you to think you could? The nagging voice within your head is holding you back – ever heard that one? Yes, we are all Spiritual Beings having a Human experience here on Planet Earth and that is the voice of the Human within us. It speaks very loudly sometimes and stops us from acting on our inner calling. Stops you from following your heart's desire and living your life full out.

It isn't that easy to listen to your heart, to stop the chatter going on in your head. Not at all. It does take practice. It is well worth the time and investment because if you are not being listened to, your body starts to build up toxins! That is unfortunately the flip side of it all – not being heard creates toxins in our system.

- What happens when your body creates toxins?
- What are some of the consequences when we allow this to occur?

Toxins create imbalance, which results in disease, illness, discomfort, pain in our body and mind. Not very beneficial for your health and vitality, and by not listening to your own inner voice, you are toxifying yourself!

- LISTEN - SILENT. The two words are spelled with the same letters. How often do you really take the time to listen within? Are you hearing, are you listening to what your heart is telling you? Your intuition?

Here is my learning lesson in life – intuition is always right. Your intuition is your Inner 'Pilot Light,' the true essence of You.

To get to hear and find your inner voice, silent space is needed, quiet time for you to just be and enjoy in stillness. Find a place where you can sit, close your eyes, and listen within.

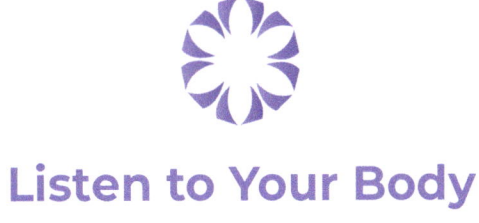

Listen to Your Body

"Everything you need to know is within you. Listen. Feel. Trust the body's wisdom."

Dan Millman

Learning to listen is a powerful tool and listening to my body has been a very rewarding journey. Our bodies are truly amazing. All the different organs and systems within, working together 24/7 to create and restore harmony for us. Did you know, our bodies always work toward balance – to restore balance so we can get on and do the things that are important for us. And when we push too hard, we knock our body out of balance and our body will tell us.

Many times, we do not listen to these 'calls.' Instead, we adapt our posture to the pain, tilt the head a bit so the shoulder discomfort isn't there; adjust our hip to avoid the back pain; and the worst thing is, we don't even notice a lot of the time.

I believe a lot of people look after their cars better than their body. Yes, the car is your vehicle that will take you from point A to B. As soon as there is an unexpected sound in the motor, we immediately drive to the service station to check it out and get it fixed, as we need the car to work properly, to move us to our physical destination. The place we want to/need to go next.

Your body is your vehicle on your Journey of Life. You can't go and just buy another body to live in. This is the one you chose for the time you have on Planet Earth. So why don't we take care of our life vehicle as well as we care for our cars?

Your body speaks to you daily. It tells you when you are too hot – you start to sweat to cool the body off. It tells you when something is wrong inside. If there is an infection, a body part will swell up, or you will get a temperature. All those small signs and symptoms, we just neglect. When we don't listen to those little signals, our body starts to scream louder. In the end it will give you more serious stuff to deal with.

Cancer, heart problems, adrenal fatigue, injuries – yes, most illnesses and injuries happen due to lack of focus and/or lack of energy. We didn't listen to the symptoms our body sent us. Then the big wakeup call comes. Fear creeps in and we finally listen and act accordingly. I believe most illnesses and injuries can be avoided, if we start to listen to our bodies a bit better. Prevention work so much better than cure!

Take a moment every morning before you jump out of bed. A moment to listen in, check out how your body is feeling before getting up and starting your day. It only takes a few minutes. Scan through your entire body, from the top of your head down to your feet and check how every little part is doing. Tune in and then give your body the love and attention it needs. Say thanks and show appreciation of your body being there for you, working well and in harmony. I am grateful for my body working so well. Do the same in the evening, after a long day's work and activities. I promise, you will sleep so much better when you give your body some love.

I have had many conversations with my body over the years. We have been through some challenges together and my mind has pushed my physical being a bit too hard sometimes. I didn't ask for permission – I just did stuff and my body didn't like it all. It comes with a price; it hurts and sometimes feelings of regret set in.

If you instead ask your body for permission and come to an agreement with your body – this is what you want to do and then move there together with your Body and Mind. Then all is well, and you give the physical attention to restore balance afterwards. If not in agreement, there will be pain and suffering. Disease a state out of ease.

Your body pays attention to you. It thinks you're important! If you've spent a whole lot of time ignoring how you feel and just bulldozing along, your body has most likely decided you're not interested in listening to these lines of communication. Your body hits the mute button. The good news is you can turn your volume back on.

> *"If you listen to your body when it whispers, you don't have to hear it scream."*
> **Source Unknown**

Listen to the Rhythms of Nature

"Life is not a mystery. It is an art we have not fully uncharted yet."

Anonymous

Eastern philosophy is based on the concept that we as human beings are an integral part of the universe. In the same way that the trees, the flowers, the clouds, and the animals are all subject to the law of nature, so are we as human beings. If we adapt and live according to the laws of nature and the changing cycles, our likelihood to live well and healthy will increase.

Everything in nature changes all the time. Nothing is completely still, there is always movement happening. Day turns to night, spring into summer, summer into autumn. All things have a birth, life and a death. Everything in nature moves according to a specific a rhythm, a cycle of its own. There are times for being active and creating, and there are times for slowing down and relaxing. Raising your awareness and moving more in tune with the natural forces around you will enhance your energy level and have you living happier and healthier.

Live with the Changes of the Seasons

> *"Springtime inspires us to believe that, along with the earth, we too might change, release the past, and give birth to new ideas."*
>
> **Madison Taylor**

Growing up in Sweden, I used to love springtime. I still do, even though the Australian weather is not expressing the change of season as clearly as back home. In Sweden, the snow melts away through the warming sun, creating the spring flood, and nature starts to wake up again after the winter slumber. I remember looking for the first signs of spring, the first little buds breaking through the earth and starting to open.

There would still be cold in the air and so much excitement around – both inside my body as well as in nature around me. This is the time to plant new seeds, time for rebirth and repopulation to fill the void of the winter. It happens every year and I still stand in awe of the new awakening taking place. Yes, excitement is in the air!

Spring is the time when we 'fall in love' again and say 'yes' to things we would normally refuse. It is the time of the year when we feel ready to try out new things, new ways of eating, new ways of exercising, new ways of being. Time to be a bit daring and start to express our inner beauty in a different way. Maybe it is that haircut that you have been thinking about for a while that will express a new facet of who you really are. Maybe it is wearing different colours; maybe it is connecting with a new group of people to build relationships with.

The energy of spring will inspire us to believe that we might change, release the past, and give birth to new ideas, new relationships, and new perspectives. Springtime encourages us to be creative, plan our future, and connect to our bigger vision and perspective on life.

Our activities should be geared towards expression of our inherent mental, emotional, and spiritual intelligence. Like we do spring cleaning of our houses and cupboards, our bodies are in action to clean up our inside both on the physical and the emotional level. Clean out the old, to allow for new to take place. In Chinese Medicine, spring is governed by our Gall Bladder and Liver energy, in charge of the smooth flow of energy throughout the body as well as storing and detoxifying the blood. Perfect time of the year to cut down on stimulants like coffee/tea and alcohol, recreational drugs, and tobacco, as nature is giving us this boost naturally through the expansive, stimulating spring energy.

Chinese Medicine also speaks about the Liver as housing the aspect of our spirit that never dies and contains our reason for being. It is said that the Liver has the capacity of determination, of bigger vision and planning, allowing us to express our greatest qualities and realise our spiritual destiny. Very strong and powerful energies that support us to face the challenges emerging from within, stop the procrastination, and allow us to move forwards with determination and clarity in mind.

Fighting the process will create imbalance within and can express itself as anger, frustration, irritation, and resentment. On the physical level there might also be aching muscles and joint pain, as Liver and Gallbladder governs our muscles, tendons, and nerves. Moving with the flow of spring energy will, on the other hand, have us express feelings of compassion, honesty, and being patient with ourselves. Patiently moving forward one step at the time towards an abundant spring filled with happiness and joy.

Summer Time

Summer, a time of the year may of us look forward to with great anticipation. The warmer weather and the sun help to improve people's mood and we are drawn outside, ready to be more active and engaged with one another. We feel full of energy and our vitality is at its peak time of the year.

Summer represents the outward moving energy, expansion, movement, and joy. Everything in nature is expressing itself, manifesting in an abundance of colours, growth, and activity. Summer is the season associated with our heart, our small intestine, and the fire energy inside our body. The heart pumps the blood to all the different organs, bringing oxygen to the cells and makes sure proper assimilation is happening in the small intestine. The small intestine is a part of our digestive system where absorption of nutrients from our food takes place. The small intestine in Chinese Medicine also has to do with how well we process and fully understand information and ideas.

This is a perfect time to nourish our spirits, realise our life potential, and connect to our inner purpose. Allow sun's nourishing energy to invigorate you and your body. We go about our work, relationships, and daily activities with a feeling of compassion, delight, happiness, and joy. When we stay connected to that feeling, we know that we are living in alignment with and are connected to nature's natural energies and rhythms.

When the heart is balanced, we feel an inner calmness and an emotional balance. A beautiful space to connect to. Unfortunately, we sometimes tend to go into excess and overdo things. Signs of this might be a feeling of nervousness, confusion, not sleeping well and being tired. It is important to stay well hydrated, eat cooling foods and getting enough sleep. Enjoy taking a nap in the middle of the day.

Yes, midday is the time of our heart energy and allowing it time to rest and recharge midday will support its function, keeping the heart energy vibrant and alive. Why not enjoy a lunch of cooling foods, followed by a 'siesta' which will also support your digestive system to get on with its work. A Healthy Habit to incorporate into your summer lifestyle. Your body will thank you for it and be so much more ready for the afternoon and evening activities.

Autumn Time - Time to Slow Down

During autumn we are moving within, getting in touch with the more serious and introspective energies associated with this time of the year. We go from the expressive and expansive energy of the summer to a more contractive and inward moving energy. It is time to slow down, time to harvest and prepare for the cooler season of winter.

Back home in Sweden, nature during autumn time offers a beautiful symphony of colours. The leaves turn red and orange before they fall off the trees, darkness sets in earlier, and the cooler air is felt both externally and internally. It is time to cultivate body and mind and become more introspective. It is also a great time for completion.

Complete and finish any project you have started earlier during the year and celebrate, enjoy your hard work. Time to let go of those things that do not serve any more. Activities, thoughts, beliefs, and relationships that are out of alignment with your bigger purpose and what you want to create in life.

Autumn time is a wonderful time to 'clear out' stuff and create space for new ideas and things to come into our life. This clearing process is not about 'getting rid of.' It's about letting go of the things and thoughts that get in the way of realising your true nature and best life.

For clearing to last, you need to change your mindset. It is a journey that does not always go in a straight line and does not always make sense. Clearing old habits and resisting behaviour is possible when you slow down. Slow down, go within, and cultivate your inner awareness of who you really are. 'Slow drip' efforts applied consistently over time is the real game changer here.

Autumn in Chinese Medicine is governed by the Lung and Large Intestine energy. This is all about exchange between our inner and the outer environment. Exchange of nutrients through the wall of the large intestine as part of your digestive system. Exchange of air through your lungs. Breathing in the nourishing fresh oxygen and breathing out the toxins, the carbon dioxide.

Exchange through the skin – the skin can be seen as an extension of your lungs. What is not discharged through your bowels or your breath, sometimes show up through the skin. Eczema, skin eruptions, boils, and pimples. This is just your body ridding itself of garbage, stuff not serving your health and future wellbeing anymore. Exchange of thoughts, feelings, and ideas through communication and expressing ourselves.

Our body is energetically in a state of letting go this time of the year. This letting go process can also show up as chest infections, flulike symptoms, or just a cold as it is governed by the Lung energy. Mucus leaving the body. Mucus filled with toxins the body wants to rid itself of.

Many of us are looking for remedies to stop this from happening, and I agree, it might not be the nicest process to go through. It is important, though, to allow your body to let go. Stopping it will only create stagnation and worsen the issues. Stay 'with the flow' and allow nature to run its natural course.

The emotion we associate with the Lung energy is the feeling of sadness and grief. If the energies are out of balance, you might feel deep sadness and have difficulty dealing with loss and any change in your life. This will weaken your lungs and if prolonged can lead to more serious problems like depression.

When we feel that inner sadness in our heart, we want to get in touch with it. Allow the grief to fully express and then 'let go,' resolving the feeling. Going through the healing process will then strengthen your Lung energy and have you more clearly been able to communicate your thoughts, to stay open to new ideas, and generally feel happier within. Letting go creates space for the new to come in.

Inability to let go can also show up as constipation. Large Intestine, the last part of our digestive system, absorbs what our body needs to function properly and releases the waste products. Often people with elimination problems will have difficulty letting go. There might also be a sense of attachment, attached to objects, people, or limiting beliefs. Emotionally, therefore autumn time is great time to look at things we might be hanging on to, work through them and then finally say 'goodbye' to them for good!

Yes, it is also a great time to let go of that extra weight you are carrying. When people come to me and say they want to 'lose weight,' my reflection on that is: when something is lost, we often go out and find it again. Rather than losing the extra kilos, entertain the idea of letting go of them. They are not needed anymore. That extra protection can go – you are working on trusting and believing who you truly are. And it is time for that shield to go.

To enhance your Lung energy, let go of negative thinking. Practice deep breathing, go outside, and breathe in the fresh morning air. Reorganise, clean up your closet, and give away all the stuff you don't need anymore – donate! Clean out your computer and your mobile phone; erase all those unnecessary contacts in there. Simplify and slow down. The activities can feel extremely liberating, lightening and are very much in harmony with natures rhythm and flow.

Hibernation time - Winter is Here

I love playing in the snow and I have great memories from my childhood of skiing to school, throwing snowballs, and building snowmen. Yes, we had proper winters, beautiful and white and yes, it was cold, and nature went to sleep, and with it many creatures in the animal kingdom. Hibernation time, time to draw inwards. Time for contemplation, inner reflection, and discoveries about ourselves.

During wintertime we are experiencing the darker, slower, inward energies of ourselves and Mother Nature. A perfect time for meditation, writing, and exercises like Tai Chi and Chi Gong.

Winter is associated with our Kidneys, which hold our body's most basic and fundamental energy. Rest is vitally important to restore, revitalise, and look after our Kidney energy, which is why some animals, as I mentioned earlier, hibernate this time of the year.

We humans should go to bed earlier and sleep longer to get the full healing benefits deep quality sleep has to offer. This is the time of the year when we need to slow down and feed ourselves both physically and spiritually. With the colder air outside, we want to feed ourselves with warmth, warming food, and powerful tonics. Learn to unplug, detach, do less and allow yourself to be a lot more. Time to be that Human Being.

> "The road to health for everyone is through moderation, harmony, and a sound mind in a sound body."
>
> **Jostein Gaarder**

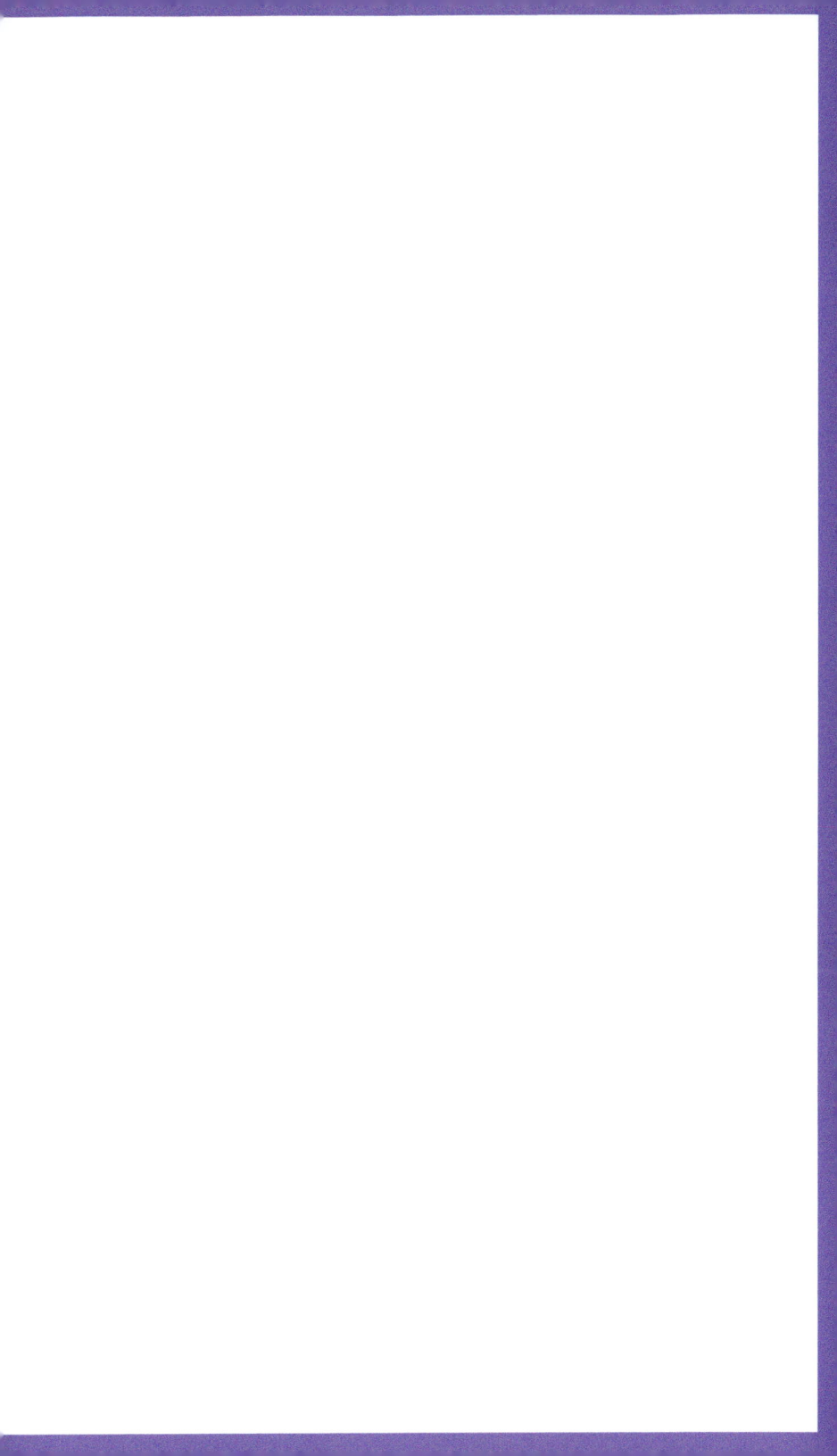

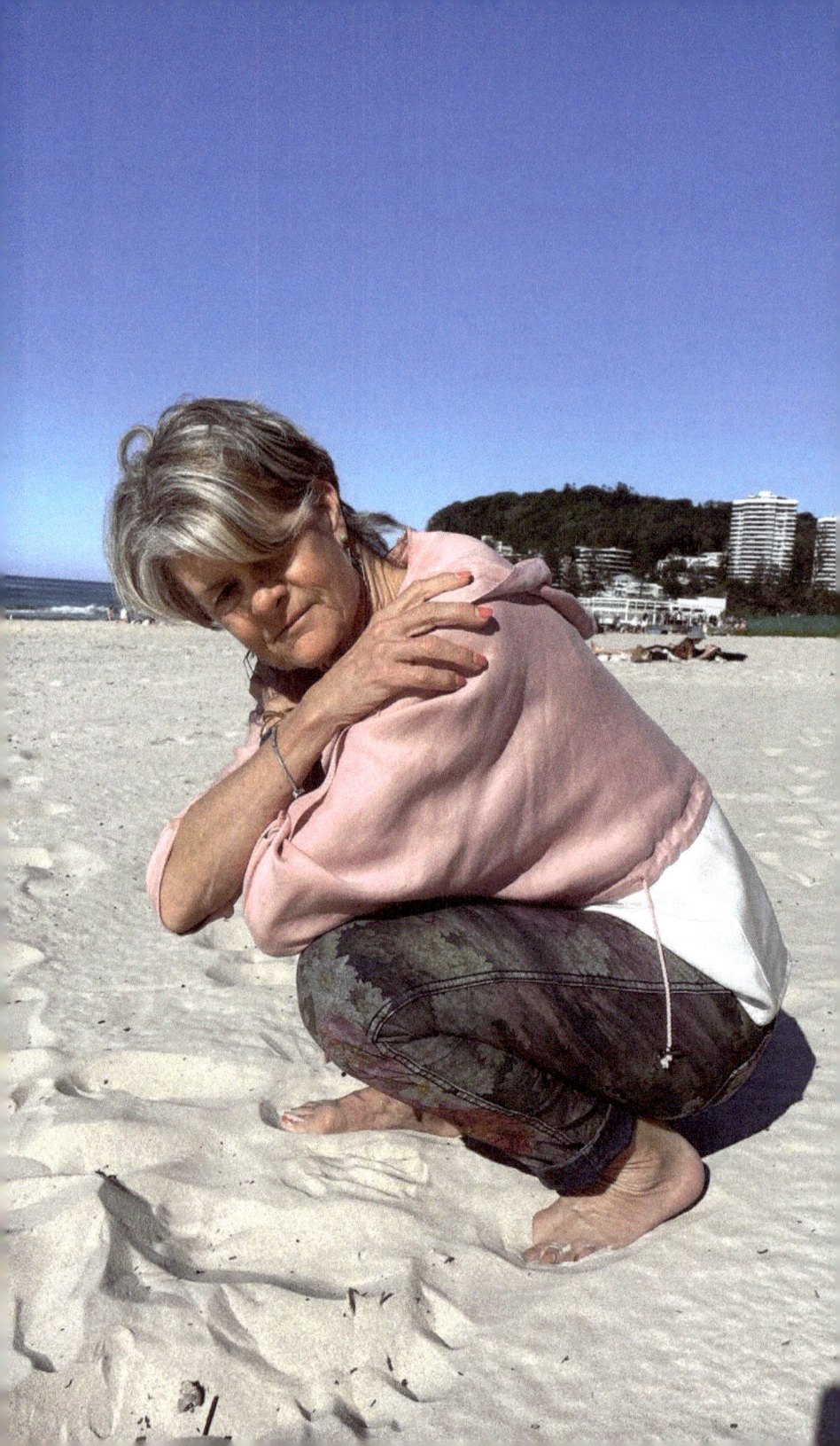

Touch

"Touch comes before sight, before speech. It is the first language and the last, and it always tells the truth."

Margaret Atwood

What a powerful quote by Margaret Atwood - and so true. Touch is the very first language we learn, already in the womb. The need to touch and be touched is established early in life as we develop and grow in the omnipresence of our mother's womb. Once we are born, separated from that sanctuary of connectivity, we begin to crave the physical embrace from others. We become more independent as we age but the need is still there. In times of challenge or when we need reassurance, a nice hug is helpful.

The most socially accepted and common form of touch is probably a handshake. A handshake can reveal quite a bit of information about the person you are connecting with if you are tuned into it – the firm, confident handshake compared to the loose or sweaty handshake you receive. Filled with information, and there are people trained in how to 'read' handshakes and gain valuable information about that person you are greeting. Coming back to Margaret's quote – touch is always true!

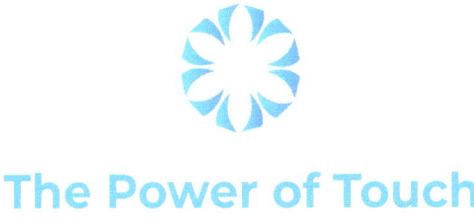

The Power of Touch

"How we underestimate the power of touch; how this one little act can break barriers, mend hearts, heal scars."

Marylin Rodrigues

Social distancing has reminded us of what a crucial role touch plays in our wellbeing. Being a tactile person, I love hugging. I love giving hugs and I love receiving hugs. In today's world, I do ask for permission to give a hug, and the interesting thing is that bodily contact is the first, endorphin-releasing language we learn as babies.

Hugging is natural, but it is also artful. Why? Because a hug must be synchronised with someone else, unlike a handshake that can be offered and accepted asynchronously.

There are studies showing that touch signals safety and trust. Touch soothes. Basic warm touch calms cardiovascular stress. It activates the body's Vagus nerve, which is intimately involved with our compassionate response. A simple touch can trigger release of oxytocin, what we also call the 'love hormone.'

Touch is the first sense we acquire and a 'secret weapon' in many successful relationships. Touch seems to be a language we instinctively know how to use, yet so many are unaware of this. Think about it – we begin receiving tactile signals even before birth, as the vibration of our mother's heartbeat is amplified by amniotic fluid.

No wonder then that touch plays a critical role in parent-child relationships from the start, and we all know it. We were never touched as much as when we are children, by our parents and others. This is when our comfort level with physical contact and with physical closeness in general develops. A crucial time for building up trust in ourselves and others.

For centuries, people have sought effective ways in which to help one another in times of need, and women have historically taken greater responsibility for caring, not only for themselves but also for others. Touch serves this purpose well – touching someone's tensed shoulders can release stress immediately, sometimes allowing tears to flow.

A release of emotions there and then and I am sure you will have experienced similar times yourself. Touch can be very healing, and it has many different applications, such a fear, anger, love, sympathy, compassion, or desire. It is the intention behind your touch that is important and the determining factor to the effect of the touch you give.

I was introduced to the greater healing benefits of touch through Shiatsu, a beautiful form of healing art derived from Japan introduced to me when I was in extreme physical pain. Yes, my body was screaming out loudly and I wanted relief from the discomfort. I was suggested to give Shiatsu a go and I am forever grateful to my friend for that recommendation. After having the course of Shiatsu treatments suggested to me, I was intrigued to find out more and went to an introductory evening to gain further information.

Timing is crucial, and this was at a time when I was ready to take charge of my own life and learn how to free myself from physical and emotional disturbances. This led me to study and later become qualified as a Shiatsu practitioner. Follow your intuition and universe provides!

Shiatsu activates the natural self-healing mechanisms of your body to instigate a change to better health. Receiving a course of regular Shiatsu treatments had me appreciate the emotional and physical strengthening within myself. I started to feel more 'alive,' vibrant, and consciously more in touch with the environment around me. I got to understand that every action I personally take will influence the whole. It enhanced my understanding of the energetic and psycho-emotional relationships of the physical structure to the mind and my emotions.

Touch is such an important part of our health and wellbeing and a wonderful way to communicate with others, sensing what is happening within.

Yes, it truly is a 'language' in itself. Our primate relatives strengthen their social bonds by grooming each other. We humans use touch to strengthen our relationships, and touch is also a marker of closeness.

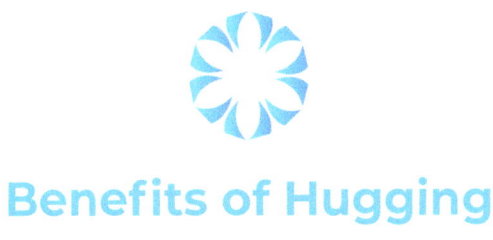

Benefits of Hugging

"A hug is always the right size."
Winnie the Pooh

Such wise word by Winnie the Pooh! I love this little bear and his wisdom.

What about hugging?! We often hug each other when we are happy or when we see the person we love most. We often feel joy and happiness when hugging another person, and a hug can convey a lot about how we are feeling and how we feel about each other. Each time we sincerely hug someone, we are conveying our love and joy for that person in a way that can never be explained through our words alone.

Since a hug requires two active participants, everyone taking part in the embrace will experience the pleasure and the joy coming from being hugged. As they wrap their arms around each other, their energy blends together and they experience a tangible feeling of togetherness. This feeling lingers long after the physical contact has been broken.

I grew up in Sweden and received plenty of hugs during my upbringing and later in life. I must admit, I love hugging and the beautiful benefits it gives me. A wonderful way to greet someone and a fantastic comforting action. And it is for FREE, with mutual benefits! Once again, the quality of the hug will reveal information about the person you are hugging. And there are so many ways to hug a person. Having said that, be daring and start hugging the people you care about. They will be happier and healthier, and it will have a positive influence on your own health at the same time:

- Hugging relaxes the body
- Hugging increases bonding
- Hugging reduces pain, as it releases endorphins in your system
- Hugging increases empathy and understanding
- Hugging alleviates stress by reducing the levels of circulating cortisol in the blood. This helps the mind to calm down
- Hugging has a beneficial influence on your heart
- Hugging improves your immune system and overall health
- Being hugged by a loved one stimulates dopamine and serotonin in your body.

If there's a most appropriate time to communicate via touch, it's probably when someone needs

Benefits of Hugging

consoling. Hugging is a wonderful way to comfort and a pleasurable way to share your feelings with someone important to you. Depending on your relationship with the other person and the message you would like them to receive, a hug can communicate love, friendship, romance, support, and any other sentiment you want to convey.

A hug communicates to another person that you are there for them in a positive way. A wonderful way to comfort someone in pain – being physical or emotional. So, please, next time you hug someone, focus your full attention on your action. That single, simple, beautiful gesture will create a profound connection with another Human Being.

There are so many ways of hugging. I have a little book called 'The Little Book of HUGS - The Complete Collection.' It is filled with various ways of hugging, from the traditional Bear Hug to the A-frame Hug, the Cheek Hug, and the Sandwich Hug. All of them have a description on how to 'perform' the hug and who it is beneficial for. The Heart-centred Hug is considered the highest form of hugging and the most beneficial for us Human Beings.

The Heart-Centred Hug begins with direct eye contact as the two huggers stand face to face with each other. You then put your left arm around the other persons shoulder and your right arm around their waist. The other person does the same. Heart to Heart! Your hearts become aligned with one another, and loving, comforting energy begins to flow between the two of you. Your souls are flooded with feelings of love, compassion, and caring. There is no time limit on this hug; it may last several moments, shutting out all nearby distractions.

The Heart-Centred Hug acknowledges that place at the centre of each of us where – if we dare to open it – pure, unconditional love may be found.

Meeting Your Own 'Needs' of Touch

"Touch the Body, Calm the Mind, Heal the Spirit"

We touch ourselves every day, without thinking about it. In the shower, washing yourself, brushing your hair, putting on body lotion, dressing and undressing. All unconscious behaviour and daily actions of touch. As I mentioned before, it is the intention of the touch that matters, so you can improve the benefits of touching yourself, by becoming more intentional about it.

When in the shower, become conscious about how you wash yourself. Have a 'conversation' with your body as you do it. Using a gentle body scrub in the morning has the added benefits of cleaning away the dead skin cells on your skin. Your body will love you for that. Wiping yourself dry with the towel is another time of touching yourself. Start doing it with love and intention. I use a spray mist and body lotion to hydrate after my shower. My intention is to give my body a bit of a massage as I do it. I rub the lotion gently into my skin, focusing my thoughts on what I am doing, soothing the muscles as I move over them with a touch of love. This does not take any extra time away in your day – just change your intention. If a body-area needs that extra bit of attention, here is your chance. You can give yourself that loving touch at any point and time in your day.

Remember, self-care is not selfish – it is essential for your future health and the wellbeing of you and others around you. Book yourself a massage and enjoy it fully once a month, if not more often. It will be relaxing, and yes, it will take time away from your daily life, but the rewards will be amazing.

Massage is a general term for pressing, rubbing, and manipulating your skin, muscles, tendons, and ligaments. Massage may range from light stroking to deep pressure. There are many different types of massage to choose between, so work out what floats your boat. You might choose a different type at different times.

Sometimes I feel the need for a deeper massage and will book myself a deep tissue massage. Other times I prefer a more gentle and soothing touch and will chose accordingly. Some people enjoy massage because it often produces feelings of caring, comfort, and connection. Try it out, connect with your body and find out what you and your body prefer, and when.

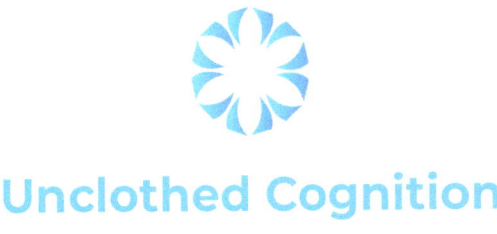

Unclothed Cognition

"Clothes make the man. Naked people have little or no influence on society."

Mark Twain

Clothes are one of the basic needs of people, along with food, water, and shelter. Growing up in Sweden, I can testify to that. My wardrobe was so much bigger than it now is. There were the clothes for summertime; for autumn and spring weather; and plenty for the wintertime with the cold weather and snow. And there were also shoes for all these different seasons. I loved my boots and I loved walking around barefoot.

I remember when we moved to the Gold Coast here in Australia. Not having worn boots for over a year and none in the cupboard, I told my husband I just had to go and buy a pair. Yep, now I always have a pair of boots available. And no, I don't have to use them for protection, but I enJOY wearing them. And it is true, it affects my mood and behaviour.

I am a small shoe size and I do have some issues with my feet. So, for me, the most important thing when I invest into shoes is comfort. I admit, they must look nice as well. Our feet carry us all day long. Yes, some of us do sit down lots and many times with shoes still on, unless you are like me, and you kick them off as soon as possible. I am the kind of person that walks around barefooted in my house most of the time. My feet love that.

It is my choice and brings me and my body lots of joy. And I love putting my bare feet in the grass or in the sand on the beach. I can remember playing in mud puddles as a young girl, enjoying squeezing the wet soil in between my toes. Pure joy and so grounding.

'Enclothed Cognition' tells us that more than its basic functions of cover and protection from the external elements, the clothes we wear have a different function. It affects us psychologically and reflects in our behaviour and thinking. This means that whatever article of clothing you wear – robes, coats, suits, onesies, masks, goggles, plastic bracelets, boots, tactical pants – can affect your thoughts and actions.

Research show that what we associate an article of clothing with has an impact on our psychology. For example, buying designer label clothing: some associate designer clothes with status and wealth, so wearing those clothes will have a specific psychological effect.

Similarly, there's also research to suggest wearing athletic wear makes us more likely to exercise; brightly coloured clothes can improve mood; and formal clothing can make us feel more authoritative and powerful. I personally know that what I dress in will affect my mood and how I feel about myself. And the clothes I wear must be comfortable – starting with my underwear. I tend to invest in natural materials that feel nice on my body. Some are more sensitive than others to the quality of the material we wear.

I also invest in good quality bedding and sheets. This is where we spend a third of our life - in bed. Going to sleep in a comfortable bed is vitally important for profound sleep and your bedding plays an important part here. I tend to like cotton – one of the most popular choices when it comes to sheets, cotton helps wick away moisture from your skin. And it feels nice and cool to my body.

Linen is another choice – wonderfully breathable and, like cotton, it wicks moisture away easily. Linen sheets keep you cool even on the hottest days. And then we have the silk option, luxurious on the skin. Silk is also a great choice if you have got allergies or skin conditions. Downside – real silk requires quite careful and attentive care.

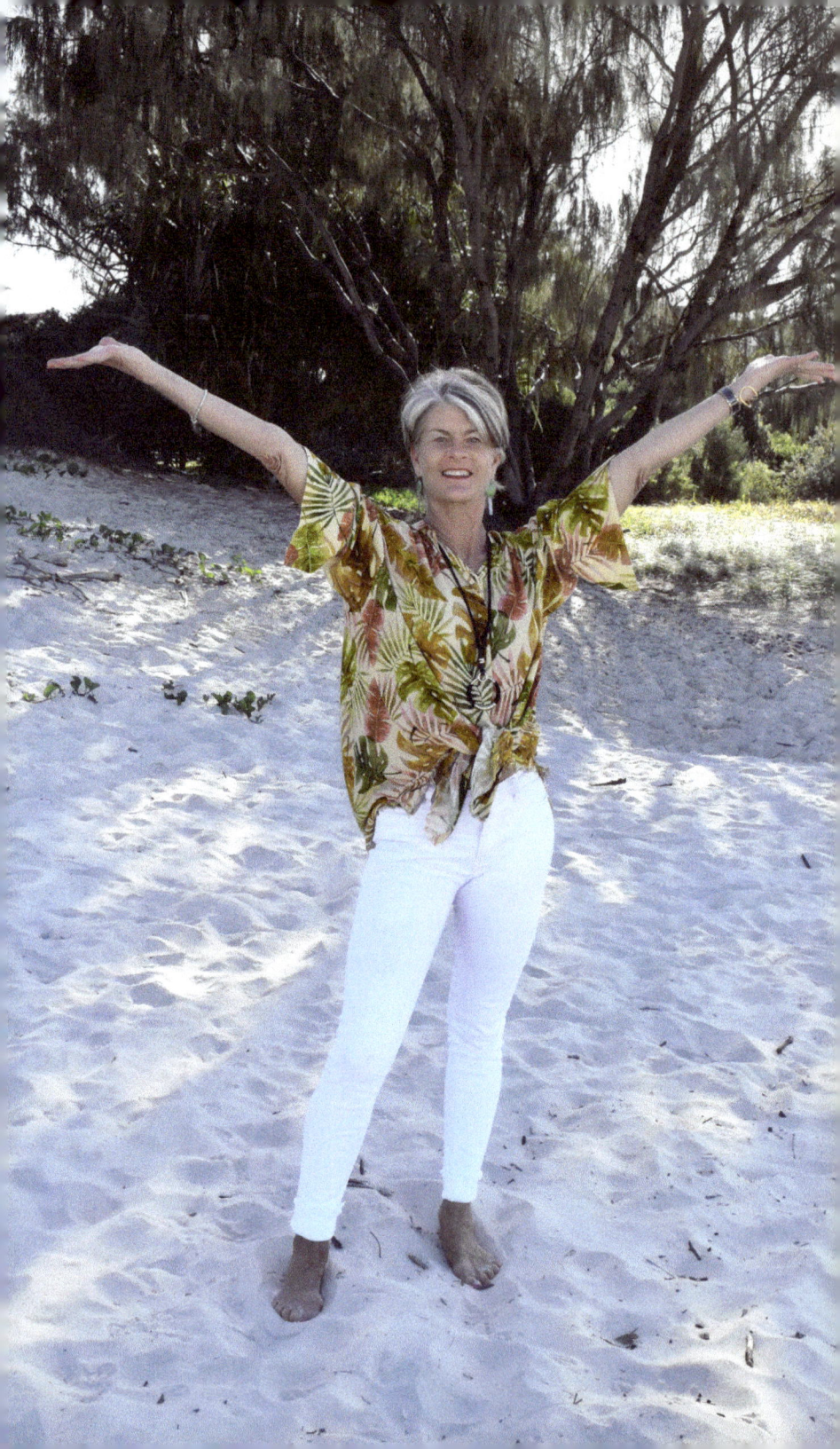

Healthy Happy Habits

"Healthy Habits are learned in the same way as unhealthy ones - through practice."

Wayne W Dyer

Unconscious Change - Embodiment

How long does it take before my new habit becomes an unconscious act, a ritual I do without thinking of having to, like brushing my teeth every morning? Research shows it takes on average 66 days for us humans to make a new habit become an unconscious ritual. This is you deciding to create a new habit, going from consciously having to think about it, to doing it automatically, without arguing with yourself, telling yourself why and how come it is important.

About two months after you made that conscious decision, you will just do it without thinking. Unconsciously. This is when you have embodied it into your mind and body. It just doesn't feel right without doing it.

Once you are there, your body will thank you for it and the future you will be a much happier and healthier you. The trick – and the challenge – is to keep your motivation up throughout the whole two months to get there. Your body helps you in the beginning. Once you made the decision your body gets a bit of a dopamine 'kick.'

Yep, the happy hormone kicks in and you feel elated just from making the decision. This will help you in the beginning. That new year's resolution is quite easy to stick to the first couple of weeks.

Unfortunately, then your body is getting used to the feeling, it is not that much fun and exciting anymore and the dopamine in your brain goes down. The stress hormone cortisol kicks in instead and you start to avoid the hard bits. A great way to keep your motivation up and trick your brain is by giving yourself acknowledgement along the way.

Set smaller goals along the way. And remember to celebrate the small successes, please. The more you do this, the more dopamine will be released and the easier to keep going. Be kind to You and your Body throughout the process and you will succeed.

This is also when your goals and intentions, your affirmations and Vision Board plays a crucial role. Please remember to read your intentions out loud every day. Your affirmation statement – 'I am…. – and look at that inspiring Vision Board of yours. Ask yourself the question: 'Why am I doing this?' The answer is right there for you – in your statements and on your board.

> *"A lack of routine is just a breeding ground for perpetual procrastination."*
>
> **Brianna Wiest**

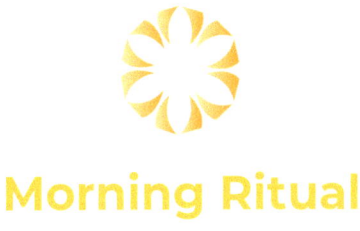

Morning Ritual

"How you start your day, is how your live your day and how you live your life."

Susanne Ridolfi

By changing your habits, you will start to change your life. As Tony Robbins so clearly states 'Willpower doesn't last, but rituals last for a lifetime.' If your goal is to step up and raise your standards, you need to back it up with rituals. I'm not asking you to incorporate all these rituals in one go. Discipline yourself in a few areas of your health and wellbeing.

Start with a couple of rituals and realise how easy it is to do those. Once you conquered a few, you start to gain momentum. You will feel the benefits and excitement in your body and mind, and you can take the next step.

Add a couple of more rituals and keep going. It is not what we get that will make us happy in life. The greatest gain in this process is who we become. And please, do not compare yourself with anyone else. You are competing with you and with what you are capable of. One step at a time and you will achieve that new standard of yours.

The Power of the Morning and a Morning Ritual

The morning is when you first download the consciousness that in many ways will dominate your day. Wisdom from ancient times teaches us that the beginning of the day is the time to think, evaluate, and correct course. As important as it is to clean and wash your body off, it is just as important to clear your mind right from the start of your day. You don't want to carry any leftover stresses from yesterday into your new day.

> *"Miracles are for everyone to write, but purification is necessary first."*
>
> **Course of Miracles**

If it is a fabulous fit body you want to create, it starts with a clean fit mind. Healthy thinking creates healthy behaviour, and your behaviour determines your result. Your thoughts affect the words you chose to use. Your words will affect your actions, which then affect the reality you create. The best time to work on this is first thing in the morning.

My own Morning Ritual is sacred. I get up before my husband and spend time with Me. There isn't a day I go without these key practices – my day wouldn't feel right without doing them. It's the same as brushing my teeth, the first thing I do in the morning. You take control of your day by taking control of your morning. You take control of your attitude and focus for the day, your energy, and your results.

Now, we are all individuals, and you will create a Morning Ritual that works for you. There are certain 'ingredients' that will be paramount to have as part of your Morning Ritual. These are called the Life S.A.V.E.R.S and were put together by Hal Elrod. The Life S.A.V.E.R.S. are simple but profound effective morning practices that will help you plan and live your life on your terms. How does that sound? Excited?

If creating a Morning Ritual is completely new to you, I suggest you start with implementing one of the practices at the time. Work on doing that single practice every morning, then add another one and then another one.

Before getting on to do your practices, please make sure to cleanse your mouth and hydrate, as described in the hydration section. To wake up the energy within and clear your energy pathways, practice the DoIn session for five minutes, as described in part 1. That will awake your body and clear your mind.

S - is for Silence.

This is your opportunity to stop, listen, and breathe. A short space of silence in the morning will help you begin the day with a calm and clear mind. It will help with your focus and what's most important. Practice the breathing meditation described earlier and you will feed every cell in your body with new fresh oxygen, energy you need to conquer and move through your day with ease and grace.

Your time in silence doesn't have to be meditation. It can also be reflections, prayers, breathing exercises. Your choice. The importance is to create a silent space, away from mobile phones and computers. For me this is quite often the beach. When I am out for my walk, I will look for a place to sit down, a place where no one will disturb me.

I will sit there quietly, listen to the sound of the ocean, and spend some time to reflect. Or close my eyes and mediate for a few minutes. For you it might be a space in your home, or out in the garden, a park, the forest. There are plenty of spaces where you can create your quiet time.

A - is for affirmation - a statement of what you want in life.

This is you programming yourself mentally. Affirmations are great for this. By repeatedly telling yourself who you want to be, what you want to achieve or create, your subconscious mind will listen and shift your behaviours and beliefs. This is what your daily affirmation is – a simple statement that defines you as you want to be, that new standard you want to raise yourself to be.

So much is happening in this world that we can't control. But life is not just about what happens, it's about who we chose to be during what's happened. The change will happen when you see the possibilities. I do this in combination with writing my morning Gratitude. I write down my daily affirmation, priming my brain to start building the belief in my mind. With consistency it will start to build that change from within. 'I am...'

V - is for Visualisation

I came across the power of visualisation the first time in university. I studied sport psychology as part of my P.E. teacher training studies and found out it was widely practised and used by top athletes. They use it to enhance their performance. Visualisation is a technique for using imagination to create what you want in life. Not only does it help you to achieve your goals and imagine your future, but also to deal with stress and so much more.

How does Visualisation work?

Visualisation works because neurons in our brains, those electrically excitable cells that transmit information, interpret imagery as equivalent to a real-life action. When we visualise an act, the brain generates an impulse that tells our neurons to "perform" the movement. The brain can't tell the difference between a vivid visualisation and the actual experience. It enables you to design the vision that will occupy your mind and making sure that the greatest pull on you is the future you want.

A great time to practice your visualisation is directly after you have done your affirmation. Close your eyes and take a few slow, deep breaths. Then start to visualise the actions you are taking for your goals/intentions to become reality. What does it look like? How does it feel? Describe it in detail – the more specific, the better, and bring in all five senses, please. How do you feel? Forget about logic and being practical. What would you have to become? When you have that clear picture in your mind, visualise yourself in total alignment with the person you must become to be there, to achieve your vision.

E - is for Exercise

If you haven't realised already, I love to move my body. This comes naturally for me and is an important part of my Morning Rituals. This is one ritual I have embodied to the point of excellence! Exercise/movement enhances your health, improves your self-confidence, and mental and emotional wellbeing. It also helps you with focus and concentration and your energy levels throughout the day. So, a vital part of your mornings.

Exercise causes the brain to release endorphins – a peptide hormone that mimics the effect of morphine. Yes, this is your natural high. The happy feelings you produce by moving your body will make it so much easier to stick to your commitments to you and your body. Moderation is the key here. Find a balance and remember – over training is as bad as under training. You will just burn out and you will not feel like exercising at all. Yep, your body will talk to you and tell you off. Listen to those signs and symptoms, please, and adjust accordingly.

So, make this a part of your morning routine, please and spend 10 - 20 minutes minimum to move. As with every little ritual, consistency is the key here as well. The benefits talk for themselves – improved blood pressure and blood sugar levels and decreased risk of all kinds of more serious illnesses like heart disease, cancer, diabetes. I have talked about this in the section about Movement, so please go back for a bit of a reminder.

R - is for Reading

This part is for your mindset, and mindset is vitally important in anything we want to achieve in life. I love reading books. I call them 'Proper' books, books I can hold in my hands. Books I can highlight things in, make notes in, and mark the bits I want to go back and re-read later. I can have a few books on the go at the same time – yes, I don't read them all from page one to the last page. I read a bit, put the book to the side and contemplate on what I read.

One of the first self-development books I read was Shirley Mac Laine's book Out on a Limb. I love Richard Bach's books and Jonathan Livingston Seagull has been read a few times by now. These are all books that lift me up and light my soul – words that have meaning and make me feel positive about life and the future. And it helps keep my mind and brain active. There is so much knowledge out there and most of it is for free.

Maybe you want to learn more about the body you live in, how it works and function. Pick up a book and enlighten yourself. Our body is amazing, and it is your vehicle in life, the vehicle you chose for this journey on Planet Earth. Knowing a few things about how it performs, and its brilliance might be useful. Who knows when that knowledge you acquired will come to use?

Try it! My hope is that you will use this book in a manner that works for you. Open the chapter that is of most value for you at this moment and time and read that. Re-read if you need and want to and let the book go, until next time you feel called to learn and get inspired.

S - is for Scribing

Scribing is simply another word for writing. This is where your journal writing comes in. I write in my Gratitude Journal every morning, as a start of my day. Now, I have committed to have this as the first thing I do, following my visit to the bathroom and grabbing my glass of lemon water. Some people journal more, some less. You just need to get started by creating the time and space for this to happen.

Scribing/writing enables you to document some of your insights and lessons learned. Write about your small successes along the way, and the bigger ones of course. How has all of this added to your personal growth and/or improvement? And there is always room for improvement.

I often ask when presenting on the topic of health and wellbeing – How are you feeling today? And, of course, I get various responses and answers. My follow up question is – Would you like to feel better? The answer is always YES! It doesn't matter if I feel fantastic already – if I could feel better, I'd say yes to that one. Wouldn't you? On top of the world – you deserve more!

Me being me, I scribe in a physical book. That's just my choice. Others choose to do their scribing digitally. In today's world, our mobile phones are used for so many things and scribing could be one of them. Please put your phone on aeroplane mode if this is your choice.

Why? You can easily be distracted by all the other stuff on your phone if you keep everything live. Yep, social media is one major disruption for us. A not so healthy habit for many and an addiction for some. So, my preferred option is a physical Journal. The choice is yours. Whatever you choose, make it work for you, please.

> *"You can't connect the dots looking forward; you can only connect them looking backwards. So, you have to trust that the dots will somehow connect in your future. You have to trust in something - your gut, destiny, life, karma, whatever. This approach has never let me down, and it has made all the difference in my life."*
>
> **Steve Jobs**

Evening Ritual

"Early to bed, early to rise, makes a man healthy, wealthy and wise."

Benjamin Franklin

Evening rituals are as important as your morning ritual. Having an evening ritual allows you to go to bed with a clear mind, sleep better, and free up space in your mind for creative thinking. Having an evening routine gives your body and mind the time and space to decompress after your active day physically and mentally. Supporting your body to a calm space and have much better sleep means you will wake up the next day feeling better rested.

I have talked a bit about this in the section on sleep. Your evening ritual is your preparation for a deep, peaceful sleep. It is vitally important that you make a conscious completion to your 'working' day. Create that action list for the next day and put it to the side.

This way you don't have to worry about it – you know what to do when you wake up. Part of this might be to slip into some comfortable clothes and decide what to wear the next day. I do this myself – I tell my husband I'm going upstairs to my bedroom to 'de-dress.' Then it is time to let go and bring your focus to your evening routine.

It might start with your evening meal. Spend a bit of time planning what to cook, then focus on the task at hand. It doesn't matter if you are on your own or cooking with someone else. Keep your focus on the meal preparation and put your heart into it. It will affect the energy in your food, and you will probably enjoy your meal in a very different way.

Evening is a great time for reflection. This can be in togetherness with your family and friends. Sharing gratitude around the dinner table is a lovely habit to create with your family. Kids love doing this and it teaches them to look at the positive parts in their day. And celebrate the small successes along the way. It is so important for children to feel they are being heard and listened to. The evening meal is a perfect time for this. I quite often ask my husband what his highlights in the day have been, as we sit down to eat together.

A nice relaxing bath before going to bed will certainly enhance relaxation. Pour a bath and put some nice smelling essential oils in there. Lavender oil is top-of-field when it comes to helping with sleep. Put the oil in the bathwater and/or on your body afterwards. If you have a diffuser, a couple of drops of lavender oil for the evening will also work well.

Lavender is also great for lowering heart rate, temperature, and blood pressure, all processes

Evening Ritual

which mirror the stages the body undergoes when easing into sleep. Lavender oil is also known to reduce anxiety. Ylang Ylang and Chamomile oils are two other essential oils with calming effects and relaxing effects on your mind.

Take time in your bath to clean your body and face. Massage some nice moisturiser into your skin afterwards and enjoy the wonderful effect your touch has on your muscles and skin. If you want to drink anything in the evening, there are plenty of nice herbal teas to choose between.

Herbal teas have long been used for relaxation and sleep, and there is scientific evidence to support herbal teas as a holistic way to reduce fatigue and improve sleep quality. Below are four different herbs that have been shown to improve sleep and promote relaxation. Try them and find out what works best for you:

1. Valerian root has a long history of being used as a sleep and stress aid. Research also shows that Valerian root is beneficial for improving sleep.

2. Chamomile has also been demonstrated to improve sleep quality.

3. Drinking a cup of Lemon Balm tea at night may reduce symptoms associated with insomnia. Lemon balm is also good for reducing anxiety and depression.

4. Magnolia bark is a traditional Chinese herb that has been used to aid sleep for thousands of years. Might not taste the best but the benefits are great.

Make a pot of tea and write in your gratitude journal to complete your day. Contemplation on the day that has been and completion of your rituals for the day. Open your windows for fresh air during the night, and please remember to turn your mobile phone off. Time for sleep, rest, and relaxation.

> *"Let her sleep, for when she wakes, she will move mountains."*
>
> **William Shakespeare**

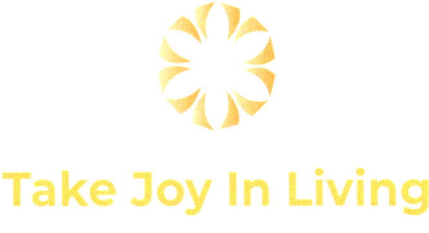

Take Joy In Living

> *"Happiness cannot be travelled to, owned, earned, worn or consumed. Happiness is the spiritual experience of living every minute with love, grace and gratitude."*
>
> **Denis Waitley**

In every given moment, you have a choice. Today I choose Happiness! Yes, that's my choice when I wake up to a new fresh day. Having read this book and taking in the ideas and guidelines for your future health and wellbeing, I wonder – what is your choice going to be? Joy is what happens to us when we allow ourselves to recognise how good things really are. So, what you choose is vitally important.

Learning how to have more joy in your life starts with your mindset. What you choose daily will set you up for the rest of that day. Match your choice with your daily routines and rituals to stay in alignment. Exercise is proven to reduce depression. Even a 15-minute run or a walk every day can boost your mood. We have together looked at finding exercise and movement you enjoy easing into making movement part of your routine. Eating right is just as important, and adding mindfulness practices like affirmations, meditation and journaling will help you feel joy daily.

We live in a fast-paced world. Always planning our next move, searching for that perfect relationship, or throwing ourselves into work and business. Social media and our phone constantly remind us of what we're missing out on. It isn't easy to keep up with everything around us and stressing about it doesn't serve. Try to 'unplug' and focus on being present to the moment. Focus on the here and now and enJOY just that.

If you're still having trouble shifting your focus to feel joy instead of negativity, try changing your posture by standing up tall. When we are challenged and feeling low and depressed, we tend to slump. Changing your posture by lifting from the top of your head, opening your chest, and taking a deep breath will help change how you feel. Confident physiology can change your entire behaviour. Bring a smile to your face. Look someone in the eyes and smile at them. You will most likely get a nice smile back – a win-win. Giving is receiving and it feels good.

> "A gentle word, a kind look, a good-natured smile can work wonders and accomplish miracles."
>
> **William Hazlitt**

The more joy you feel, the more you will attract joy in your life. This is how the Law of Attraction works. A principle that has been around for thousands of years and is still used by the world's most successful people to design the lives of their dreams. You can too. It is very simple: what you focus on, you attract. When you choose to focus on creating joy in your own life and sharing it with others, you will naturally attract even more joy.

The same goes with the people you choose to hang out with. When you surround yourself with uplifting, positive people you attract more of the same. Fun, excited people that enjoy life and lift your spirit. They will help you find the good things in every situation. Yes, this sometimes means letting go of some so-called friends. If that relationship isn't in alignment with what you want to achieve in life, you might be better off without it. Remember, it is important to let go to give space for new to come in.

Contributing to a good cause is something that brings joy into my life. Some will say that the secret to living, is giving. Now, giving back does not have to be about money or physical things. You don't need money to find fulfilment through giving. You can donate your skills, your expertise and time to a good cause. I believe time is the most valuable 'thing' we can give to others. Time is something you never get back. A listening ear can be enough sometimes. When you practice 'empowered listening,' you are providing a healing space for your partner. Practice the art of giving and find that you are making a difference in the life of others. You just need a desire to do good in the world and be willing to donate.

> *"Life isn't about getting and having, it's about giving and being."*
> **Kevin Kruse**

Get Ready for Takeoff - It is Time to Thrive

> *"I am the master of my fate;*
> *I am the captain of my soul."*
>
> **William Ernest Henley**

Get ready for takeoff! It is time to stop living in the past. Time to unleash your ultimate health and vitality and start being the vibrant woman you so deserve. It is my hope that this book will inspire you and help you achieve your intentions and goals about Your Body and You.

Please go back to the sections that speaks most loudly to you and start there. When you listen to your body, you will know which areas are in need right now. That's where you start and look at creating a small ritual to nurture that part of you that is lacking. Gradually create sacred rituals that work for you and help create the changes you want to see and experience. Remember - willpower doesn't last, but rituals last for a lifetime!

Build momentum and start to take control today, tomorrow, and for the years to come. What we practice we embody, what we embody we become. Awaken and become - sustainable energy, radiance, and wellness is what you want and so deserve. Why not create a life as joy-filled and fulfilling as the one you dream about? Listen to what Marianne Williamson so beautifully says:

> "Our deepest fear is not that we are inadequate. Our deepest fear is that we are powerful beyond measure. It is our light, not our darkness that most frightens us.
> We ask ourselves - 'Who am I to be brilliant, gorgeous, talented, fabulous?'
> Actually, who are you not to be?"

Bibliography

Books:

'Out on a Limb' - Shirley MacLaine

'You Can Heal Your Life' – Louise L Hay

'The Power Of Now' – Eckhart Tolle

'You Can't Afford The Luxury of a Negative Thought' – John Roger & Peter Williams

'Power Vs Force' – David R Hawkins

'Have You got the GUTS To be Really Healthy?' – Don Chisholm

'The On Purpose Person' – Kevin W McCarthy

'The Magician's Way' – William Whitecloud

'One Bite At A Time' – Sarah Lantz & Tanita McIntosh

'Go Girl' – Natalie Cook

'The Aging Myth' – Joseph Chang

'SHIATSU' (The New Life Library) – Susanne Franzen

'Shiatsu For Women' – Ray Ridolfi & Susanne Franzen

'The Healthy Home' – Gina Lazenby

'The Lagom Life' – Elisabeth Carlsson

'Zen Mind, Beginners Mind' – Shunryu Suzuki

'Listen – there is a world out the waiting to be heard' – Carol McCall

'The Alchemist' – Paulo Coelho

'Jonathan Livingstone Seagull' – Richard Bach

'Illusions' – Richard Bach

'The Five Minute Journal' – Intelligent Change

'Daily Mantras To Ignite Your Purpose' – Lisa Messenger

'The Little Book of HUGS' - the complete Collection' - Kathleen Keating

About the Author

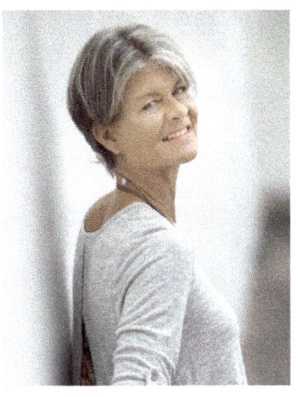

Susanne Ridolfi is a Health Coach, Speaker & Author who has been involved with Oriental Medicine for over 35 years.

Originally from Sweden, Susanne started her career as a physical education teacher. She represented Sweden as a teenage gymnast, has trained in dance, worked as a Personal Trainer, and coached gymnastics teams. Her educational background also includes university studies in Psychology and Sociology.

Following her interest in integrative medicine, Susanne trained in Shiatsu-Do, Tai Chi, Chi Gong, and Do-In. She is also a Cranio-Sacral therapist and coaches in Listening and Communication skills.

In 1989, Susanne became Co-Principal of the British School of Shiatsu-Do based in London. Together with her husband, Ray, she set up a network of franchises throughout UK and travelled across Europe to teach and lecture in the areas of Shiatsu, health, and wellbeing.

In 2002, Susanne moved to Australia with her family. She now lives in Burleigh Heads on the Gold Coast where she operates her wellness business. Susanne is dedicated to supporting ordinary people to create extraordinary lives for themselves and their families.

She is the founder of FEMALE Entrepreneurs MeetUp group, a networking community based on the Gold Coast. The community is a wonderful tribe where women come together to be inspired, grow, and to connect with like-minded spirited women.

Her mission is to inspire women around the world to enjoy an abundance of energy and a deep connection with the body they live in through cultivating a culture of self-care.

She is the author of several acclaimed books:

'Shiatsu For Women' (co-author with Ray Ridolfi)

'Guide to Natural Therapies' (author of chapters on Shiatsu and Do-In)

'The New Life Library, Shiatsu '(author)

To find out more information about Susanne, log on to:

www.susanneridolfi.com

www.ingramcontent.com/pod-product-compliance
Ingram Content Group UK Ltd.
Pitfield, Milton Keynes, MK11 3LW, UK
UKHW061223180426
11947UKWH00027B/1994